"Homework?
My Locker Ate It!"

An Effective Method for Parents to help Their Student Study at Home and Improve in School

---

Ross Quackenbush, Psy.D.
Jerrel Gastineau, M.S.Ed.

COUNSELING AND WORKSHOP PROFESSIONALS
965 Ewald Avenue S.E.
Salem, OR 97302
Telephone: (503) 588-1010

Copyright © January 1, 1988 by Dr. Ross Quackenbush and Jerrel Gastineau, M.S.Ed.. All rights reserved. No part of this book may be reproduced in any form, electronic or mechanical, including photocopy, recording, or any information storage and retrieval system without permission in writing from the publisher, Counseling and Workshop Professionals.

The front cover was illustrated by Darlene Thiesies. The rest of this book was written and illustrated on a Macintosh SE 20 megabyte hard drive computer by Dr. Ross Quackenbush in collaboration with Jerrel Gastineau, M.S.Ed..

ISBN 0-9621701-0-0

To Beth, Kelly and Brian who make it all worthwhile.
R.A.Q.

To Corrina and my kids.
J.L.G.

CONTENTS

INTRODUCTION _____ 1

Help Is On The Way! _____ 3

WEEK 1, *Getting Organized* _____ 7

WEEK 2, *You Can Improve On Last Week* _____ 23

WEEK 3, *Shaping Behavior* _____ 43

WEEK 4, *Feeling More Confident* _____ 56

WEEK 5, *Thinking Positive* _____ 72

WEEK 6, *The Value Of Organization* _____ 92

WEEK 7, *Staying With It* _____ 110

WEEK 8, *The End Of The Beginning* _____ 124

Appendix A, *Certified Leaders* _____ 137

Appendix B, *Extra Forms* _____ 138

Appendix C, *Advanced Achievement Ideas* _____ 142

Introduction

Jerry Gastineau, M.S.Ed. and I have developed a successful method to *help underachieving students* that we call the **Academic Skills Workshop.** It was designed to help middle and high school students who are getting "D" and "F" grades improve their academic performance.

Although the book was designed to meet the needs of failing students, *students need not be failing to benefit greatly from this book.* In fact, we hope many users will be parents and students who simply want be sure the student is developing first class study habits - the kind of learning habits that promote self-esteem, autonomy, and self-confidence.

The practical advice you will find on these pages comes "hard earned" after 5 continuous years of **Academic Skills Workshops** that we have done with parents and students. We think parent involvement is so crucial that we *insist* the parent come if they want help for their child. This workshop is demanding, but richly rewarding work; few experiences in counseling are more exhilarating than watching previously failing students learn to believe in themselves and to see their parents become proud of them.

You might wonder if it is necessary that your child "wants" to learn to study better. Quite frankly, we think many of you will be able to help your child, even if they are initially resistant and don't want to do it. Some students ask their parents to come to our workshops, but many are initially scared and resistant. *That's understandable; underaching students know this is a weak area and would prefer to avoid adult attention if possible.* However, the plain truth is that only a small minority of failing students learn to achieve without structured adult help. Most caring parents cannot passively stand by while their children "go under." We think that developing strong study habits in children is a challenging, high level parenting problem.

We also think that after the ability to love self and others, it is one of the greatest lasting gifts parents can give their children.

From the first chapter, parents will learn how to:

* respond when your *underachieving child* tells you he/she "doesn't have any homework." (!)
* structure your child to study 5 nights a week and turn in assignments.
* have your student collect valuable information about how much time he/she actually spends **on-task** on each subject.
* use a simple method to get feedback from the teachers before it is too late.

We wish you well on your *important journey* and sincerely hope to meet you again for a chat on the other end of the book!

Dr. Ross Quackenbush   Jerry Gastineau, M.S.Ed.

Counseling and Workshop Professionals
965 Ewald SE
Salem, OR 97302
(503) 588-1010

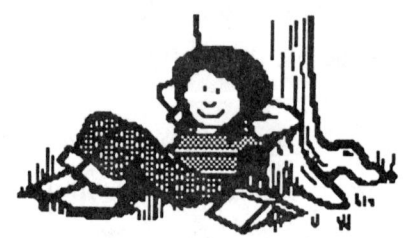

(Teachers, Counselors, and Principals who are interested in learning an inexpensive group method to involve parents in their child's education may wish to contact us about training/materials for the ACADEMIC SKILLS WORKSHOP.)

Help is on the way!

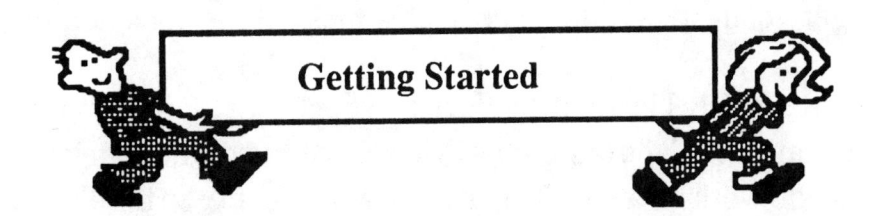

Getting Started

The Case of the Absent Mind

I was puzzled. My soon to be partner, Jerry Gastineau, M.S.Ed., had referred Jack to me for evaluation, and I didn't know why he was getting "D's" and had failed several courses earlier in the year. Jack was in the 9th grade and had an I.Q in the top 10% of the population. He read well, had good comprehension, and attended school regularly. There were some family problems but he wasn't being abused. It seemed to me that he shouldn't get less than a "C" in anything if he just sat there.

Jack Had Taken a Serious Dive:

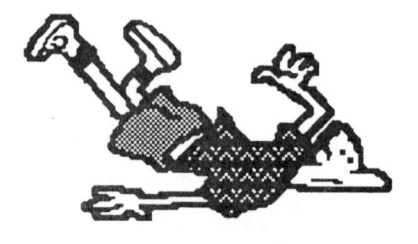

Potential = Top 10%
Grades = Bottom 10%

I was in graduate school and was studying about 40 to 50 hours a week in addition to going to classes and doing part-time counseling. I didn't know I could work so hard. Jack wasn't working at all. Personally, it bothered me that such a bright youngster could make such a mess of his considerable gifts.

As I listened carefully I learned that Jack had honed his "failure skills" to a sharp edge. He usually didn't do assignments in school and he didn't take work home. When he did do work he often "lost" it somewhere between his class, locker and home. He couldn't seem to find his books. However, he was a "good sport" about it all, and, when pressed, he said he was willing to work harder but, unfortunately he couldn't because, *"he didn't have any homework."* When I heard this, half of me was filled with the admiration one feels for a true artist in his chosen field. However, the other half of me was deeply touched by his denial that he had a problem at all. We decided to make his study habits the first priority.

Fortunately, if there was one thing I knew how to do, it was to study. After considerable thought, I decided to approach this problem by making a plan to change his behavior first, because *it didn't seem possible to change the way he thought about it,* just yet. The first thing was to tell him that **there is no such thing as not having homework, and make it stick.** We bought him an

4

inexpensive stopwatch and I taught him to record **on-task** study time. Next, we negotiated with him that 15 minutes a night was a reasonable amount of time to study (remember - he didn't study at all in the beginning). To help with having enough homework, Jack was instructed to tell each of this teachers that he was going to study 15 minutes every night and *"could they please help him out?"* (the teachers were most gracious and enthusiastic about it). We charted his progress and he kept an assignment sheet. After 7 weeks he had slowly worked up to 60 minutes of **on-task** time per night.

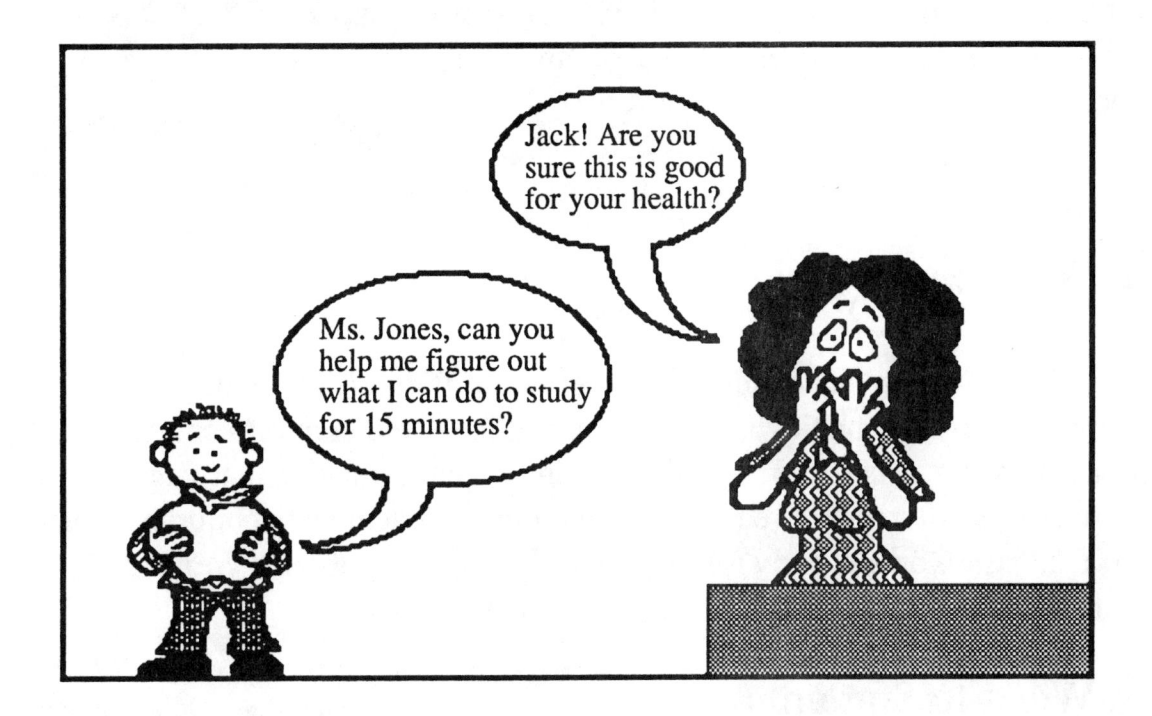

> Ms. Jones, can you help me figure out what I can do to study for 15 minutes?
>
> Jack! Are you sure this is good for your health?

The result was gratifying. At the end of the quarter, his GPA in academic subjects improved from a D+ to a C+. Furthermore, *in every prior quarter* he had been marked down in the comments section of his report card for "does not turn assignments in on time." This time two of his teachers marked "positive class attitude" and for the first time none of his teachers marked that he *didn't turn assignments in on time*. Though still not functioning at his true potential, Jack and his parents were pleased.

As a side effect of Jack's effort, **the conflict level at home over school decreased** considerably. Summer came and we discontinued counseling.

A Note of Caution

In December, I got a call from Jack's mother. He was failing again. I asked her,

"Are you still following the Study Plan?"
She said, "Study Plan, what Study Plan?"
I said, **"You know,** the Study Plan we worked so hard to get started."
She said, "Oh, the **STUDY PLAN.**"

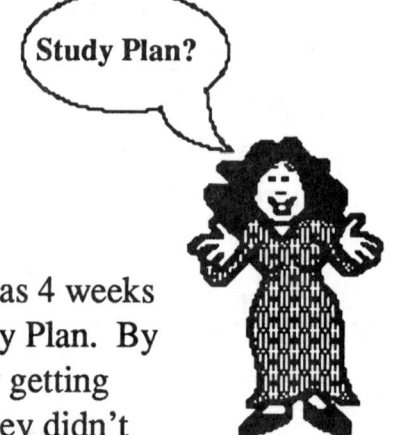

I told her the next Academic Skills Workshop was 4 weeks away but to get started *right away* on the Study Plan. By the time the Workshop started Jack was already getting mostly "A" and "B" feedback from teachers; they didn't really need the workshop. **What they needed was parent follow-through.**

A Word to Parents

Positive change in our children is sometimes difficult (but not impossible) to sustain. Enter this book with hard love, soft love, and commitment. You will not find short cuts. You **will find** an intelligent structure that can make a remarkable difference. We think that helping underachieving children learn to do academic work properly is a **high level parenting problem.** We need to join with your parenting skills to help your student.

A Word to Students

Although this is a book about study skills (with pictures, stories and a little humor thrown in), it really has a much deeper message "between the lines." Among the greatest gifts you can give yourself and your parents, is the full use of your own mind. **Let us help you. This is not the time to be contrary!**

If you understand this book, you will see that we want you to be **stronger** and **more in control** of your life. Our best wishes are with you.

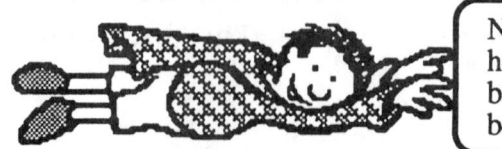

Week 1

Getting Organized

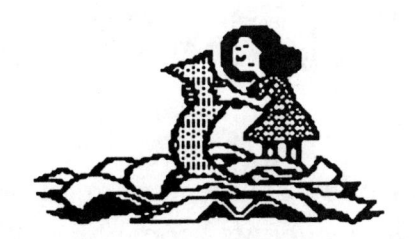

How to Use This Book

This is a method for the **parent and student to work together.**

It assumes a caring relationship exists between the parent and student. If you are experiencing high levels of conflict we recommend you check the list of counselors trained in this method in Appendix A to see if one is near you before starting. You may also wish to call this counselor if you get "stuck" later. Sometimes people need someone to help them make changes. If a counselor trained in this method is not available, go to the counselor at school or find one in private practice. The point is, if you are not able to do this book on your own, **don't stop, get help.** If things between you are OK, please continue.

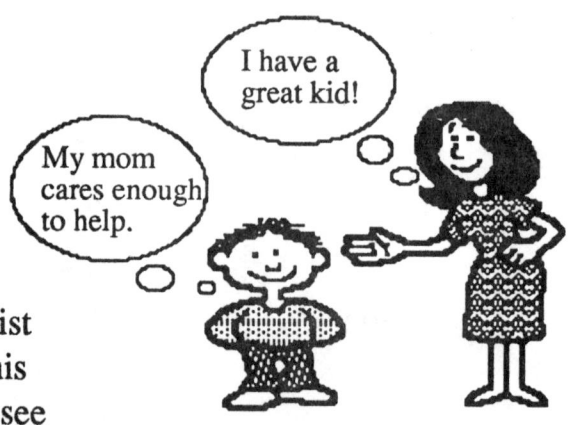

Each section is designed to be **read by the parent first.** The student reads the chapter next. However, in some cases, it may work best for the parent to simply explain it to their student. Parents know their child best and must be the judge of this.

We wrote this book because few things in our counseling experience give us more pleasure than watching students "come alive" and begin to show their potential. Common "side effects" of better study habits are a rise in self-esteem, less tension at home in the evening, and better communication.

This method focuses on the **joint responsibility** of the parent and student to help change study behavior. Poor study skill should be viewed as an important parenting challenge. In our experience, the rate of "spontaneous recovery" is very low. With rare exceptions, students who begin to slide usually continue without adult help. In most cases, **active home support is the only possible answer** Using our method, this will often be successful.

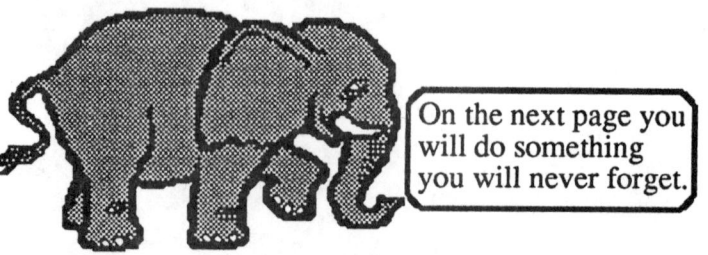

On the next page you will do something you will never forget.

Contract

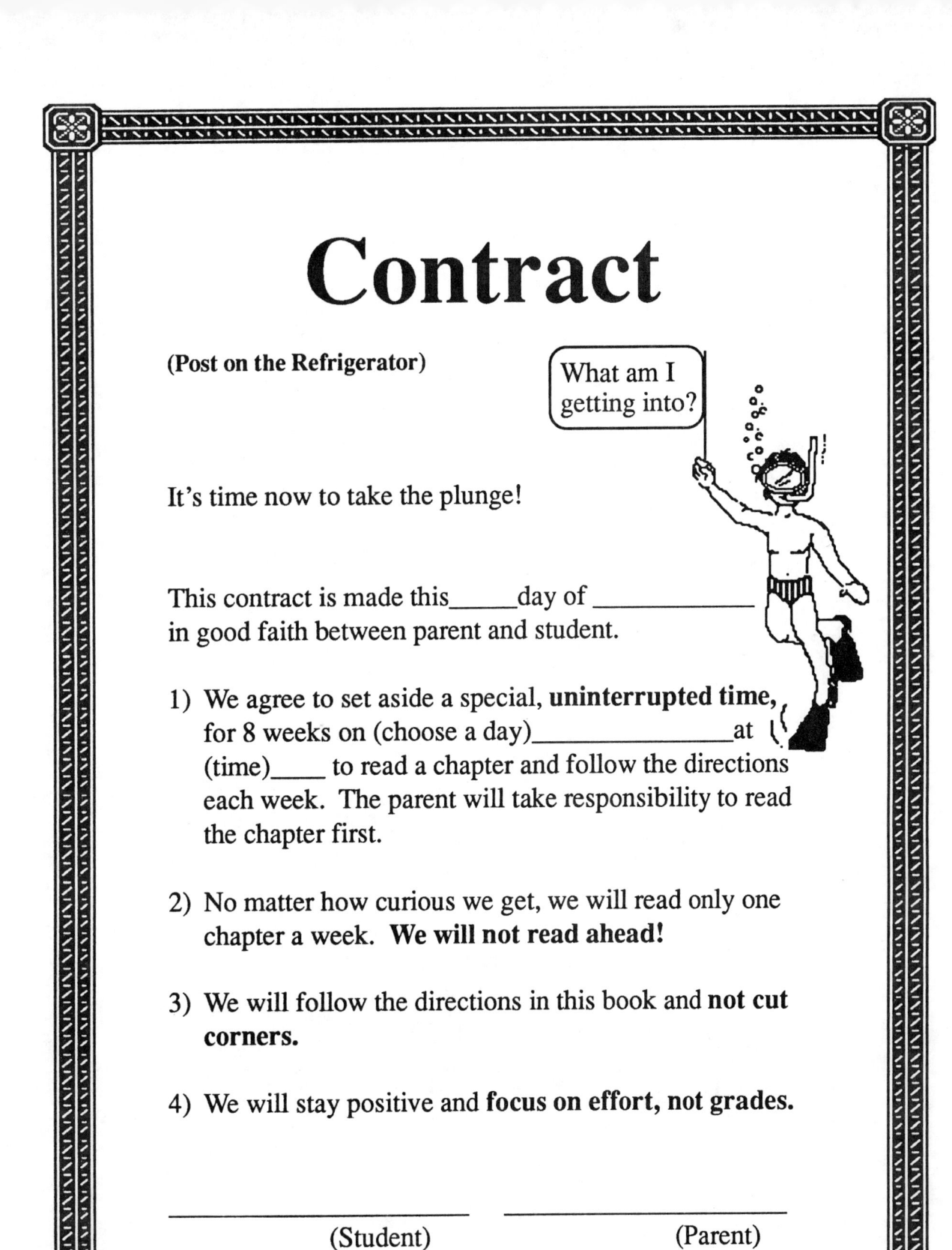

(Post on the Refrigerator)

What am I getting into?

It's time now to take the plunge!

This contract is made this_____day of _____ in good faith between parent and student.

1) We agree to set aside a special, **uninterrupted time,** for 8 weeks on (choose a day)_____at (time)____ to read a chapter and follow the directions each week. The parent will take responsibility to read the chapter first.

2) No matter how curious we get, we will read only one chapter a week. **We will not read ahead!**

3) We will follow the directions in this book and **not cut corners.**

4) We will stay positive and **focus on effort, not grades.**

_____   _____
(Student)   (Parent)

Remember to **Post** this!

The Study Plan

On the next few pages you will learn the most important skill in the entire book: how to focus your attention. Please pay close attention and do things **exactly** as we explain them.

Do not take shortcuts!

We will now direct your attention back and forth between pages. Please just follow along. When you understand what we have explained it will be **quite simple.** At first, it may appear complicated, but after a little close attention, it will be very, very easy (this is often true of school books too!).

Now look at the next page. It says **Study Plan** at the top. Students are to **carefully tear out the Study Plan along the perforation and put it in the front of your notebook.** ◁ Do it now ▷

Write your name and date in the top right spaces provided. Next, write *all* of your school subjects (except P.E.) in the left hand column where it says "subjects." ◁ Do it now ▷ Briefly look over the rest of the chart and then return to this page.

Some of you may have guessed that the student will be **recording important information** about him or herself. You were right! Continue on.

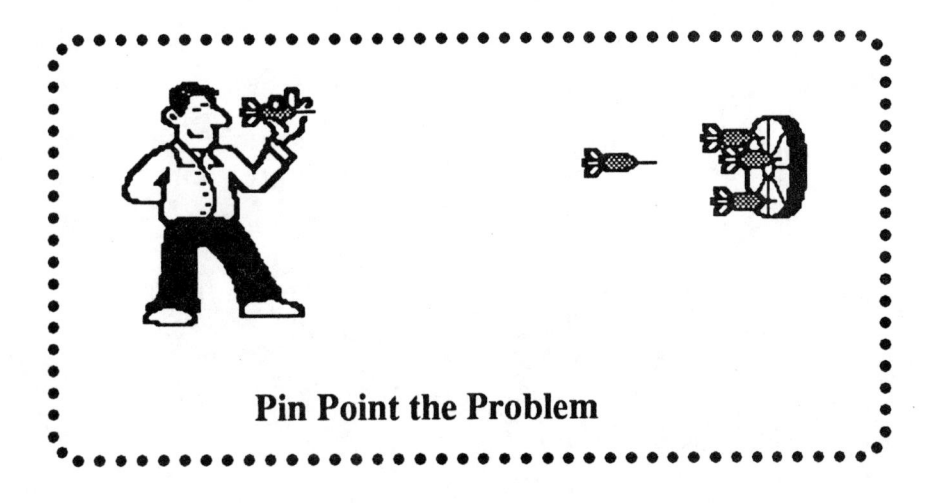

Pin Point the Problem

Study Plan
Academic Skills Workshop

Name: _____

Date: _____

Daily Goals

Subjects:							Week Total	**Teacher Comments:** Grade/Attitude/All Work Turned In?

Total Stopwatch Time For All Subjects:

When Did You Start?
When Did You Finish?

Place You Studied:

Parent's Initials:

WEEKLY AVERAGE = _____ Minutes/Day
(Add total number of minutes for the week and divide by 5 days.)

COPYRIGHT © January 1, 1988 by Counseling and Workshop Professionals

Unauthorized Reproductions Are Illegal and may be Punishable by Large Fines.

Students who have individually purchased this book may make copies for their own personal use. Copies may not be made for friends. School Districts are **Expressly Forbidden** to replicate these materials. A special discount is available to schools. Call (503) **588-1010** for ordering information.

Now look below. You will see a miniature study plan with 3 subjects listed (you will probably have 5 or 6). Notice those **odd little lines in "mid air"** that are in the top row underneath the **Daily Goals** heading. Underneath the first line on the left, the student writes the **day of the week** it is today, and then fills in the rest of the days of the week, in order, across the page. Look at the example below, and then turn back to your chart and fill in the weekdays. ◂ Do it now

When you are done, the top of your chart should look like the one below except our student (Kevin) has written 30 (for 30 on-task minutes he will study that day) across the top of each line too, and crossed out the 2 days he will take off during the week.

STUDY PLAN
Academic Skills Workshop

Name _Kevin_
Date _10/8/88_

Daily Goals

("mid air" lines) →

Teacher Comments: Grade, Attitude, Work in?

Subjects:	30 W	30 Th	~~F~~	~~S~~	30 S	30 M	30 Tu	Week Total	
English	20	15			20	20	20	95	
Math	0	0			0	5	0	5	
Social Studies	10	15			10	10	5	50	

Total Stopwatch Time

Start/Finish

Place You Studied

Parent Initials

Weekly Average=____
(Add total number of minutes for the week and divide by 5 days.)

On your chart, leave the number of minutes you will study blank for now (parent and student will negotiate this later in the chapter). However, students, **you should now decide which 2 days you want off** and mark a line through them now like Kevin did. **You must study the other 5 days.** ◂ Do it now

It may have seemed odd to start a week in the middle (for example, it may have been Wednesday) but we are going to keep track of exactly one week at a time so we must start on the day you actually began (today).

12

Using Your Stopwatch

Each student **must have a stopwatch** (this is important, *please don't use a regular clock*). We use it to keep track of **on-task** study time which we will record in your chart. **On-task time** is quite different from how long the student sits at a table or desk. Students, not parents, use the stopwatch.

> **The stopwatch rule is simple: run the stopwatch only when you are ACTUALLY PAYING ATTENTION to doing your homework.**
> **This is on-task time.**

You must turn it off immediately when you:

* Are interrupted for any reason (even by your parents, brothers, or sisters).

* Go to the bathroom or get something to eat.

* Find your mind is wandering or you daydream about anything (even if it's that you don't want to do homework!)

* Are not actually paying attention to your homework for *any* reason.

There are many excellent reasons why you must use the stopwatch in this way. To begin with, many students like the fact that when they have reached the amount of study time they contracted for, they can be done. (Of course they may study longer if they like, but they are agreeing to a minimum at this point.) We like the reason that the stopwatch actually functions as a **biofeedback tool** that tells students when they are really working and when they are not (and it never yells, scolds, nags, or loses it's patience!). There are other reasons too, and for these we look again at Kevin's chart. After he has worked on this plan for one week his chart is filled in as shown on the next page.

Completely filled in chart:

STUDY PLAN
Academic Skills Workshop
Daily Goals

Name **Kevin**
Date **10/8/88**

("mid air" lines) →

Teacher Comments: Grade, Attitude, Work in?

Subjects:	30 W	30 Th	? F	? S	30 S	30 M	30 Tu	Week Total	Teacher Comments
English	20	15			20	20	20	95	A-, Great Attitude! ALL ASSIGN IN
Math	0	0			0	5	0	5	F, lousy ATTITUDE 10 ASSIGN BEHIND
Social Studies	10	15			10	10	5	50	B, GOOD ONE ASSIGN LATE
(Daily Stopwatch time in each subject) ↑↑ et.									
Total Stopwatch Time	30	30			30	30	30	150	Weekly Average = **30.0**
Start/Finish	6:30/7	6:15/6:45			6:30/7	6:15/6:45	6:30/6:45		(Add total number of minutes for the week and divide by 5 days.)
Place You Studied	Table	Table			Table	Table	Table		
Parent Initials	RQ	RQ			RQ	RQ	RQ		5)150

Notice that Kevin, like you, is required to study 5 days a week. He took Friday and Saturday off. Next, look below the heavy black line and see that he added up all the time he studied each day (30 minutes) and wrote it where it says Total Stopwatch Time on his chart. Likewise he wrote the time he **started and finished** his homework on the chart, the **place where he studied,** and he got his **parent's initials** every night. Each day, you (the student) are to do the same on your chart. Be sure you understand this before you go on. (Parents, we expect your student to bring you the Study Plan each night. However, if your student does not bring you the **Study Plan,** ask for it.)

Kevin takes his plan to all his teachers once a week:

After he studied for a week he **took his Study Plan to all his teachers** (since he started on Wednesday, he got his feedback on Tuesday the following week). If for some peculiar reason he would have "forgotten" he would have done it the next day or until he "remembered". **You are to do this too,** and of course you would never "forget" such an important task.

Hint: Teachers appreciate getting your Study Plan at the beginning of the period.

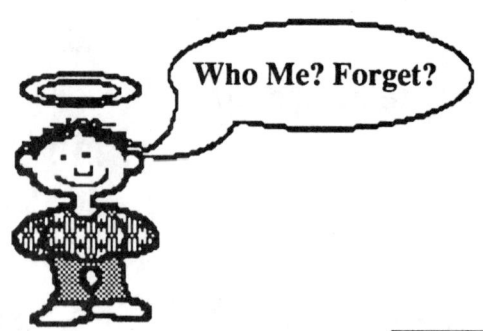

Who Me? Forget?

Students: you are to get feedback on your chart from all your teachers once a week. Together with your parent, pick a day to do this. ◀ Do it now

The information that Kevin collected with his stopwatch has become quite valuable to know how to help him. If you look in the Week Total column you can see exactly how much he studied in each subject. Perhaps one or two parents out there in readerland noticed that he is failing in math. It may also have occurred to our more perceptive readers that he might be failing because, other than on Monday, when he was truly "inspired" to study math for 5 minutes, he is **avoiding** math.

> **When students (or adults) avoid doing difficult, but necessary things, they are often in unconscious denial they have a problem. Typically, they make up excuses that sound absurd to other people but have the effect of blocking change.**

We will tell you how to use this information in later chapters. For now, simply note that by charting we see a pattern of avoidance that was causing him to fail.

That's the basics and it is really simple.

Now you know about **on-task time** and how to record it. At this point, the parent and student are to take a few minutes to negotiate how much time the student will study 5 nights a week and write it above the line in "mid air." Pick an amount of time that **you know the student can achieve** (with "former nonstudiers" you should not start higher than 20 minutes/night) so you will have success. Remember, you will be following this plan for 8 weeks and will have the opportunity to gradually add more time each week until the student is studying between **60 and 90 stopwatch minutes** per night. ◀ Do it now

Do Not Proceed Until You Have Done This!

The Assignment Sheet

In addition to recording stopwatch time, the student must record one more thing: the assignments given in school. On the next page is the Assignment Sheet. Look at it now. It is very simple. The student is to write down the **exact assignment before leaving each class, and the dates of any tests and quizzes** they are going to have. There is a space for the name of the class, what the assignment is, the date it was given, the date it is due (even if it's the next day), and most importantly, the date the assignment was **actually turned in** (hopefully this will be the same as the date it was due!) A sample is shown below:

Assignment Sheet

Write down the exact assignment before leaving class

Class	Assignment	Date Given	Date Due	Date Turned In	Parent Initial
English	Chap 7, 65-71	10/9	10/10	10/10	RQ
Math	Chap 4, 46-48	10/9	10/10	10/10	RQ
S.S.	Chap 6, 54-58	10/9	10/10	10/12*	RQ
Math	TEST COMING!	10/10	10/14	10/14	RQ
English	QUIZ	10/11	10/11	10/11	RQ

Now, **tear out the assignment sheet** on the next page of this book and put it in *front* of your Study Plan in your notebook and start recording all of your assignments, starting today. ◁ Do it now

Parents, please help your student follow-through with this. For many students, this is **more important than the amount of study time they do!** If your student has "trouble remembering" then it will help if you put your initials in the last column **each night** after asking if all assignments were written in. Don't be in a hurry to get a quick answer. If you take your time over the answer, you may help your student remember things he/she had forgotten.

16

Assignment Sheet

Write down the exact assignment before leaving class

Class	Assignment	Date Given	Date Due	Date Turned In	Parent Initials

SECTION SUMMARY: So far, you have learned how to do 3 main things, (1) how to record on-task time, (2) get feedback from your teachers every week, and (3) keep an assignment log. There is one more critically important issue to deal with; the student agrees to follow this plan but wants to know "what do you do if you don't have any homework?" Not many adults know the only correct answer to that question but we do. The only correct answer answer is: **There is NO SUCH THING as not having homework!** This possibility **simply does not exist.** We'll tell you why:

WHY THERE IS NO SUCH THING AS NOT HAVING HOMEWORK

Using your mind 5 nights a week is **not optional.** We know from experience that the only students who say they "don't have any homework" are either <u>failing</u> or <u>underachieving</u>. The fact is, when we hear this, we *know it simply means the student has a serious problem.* However, if you think you don't have homework you are to do the following:

1) You have our **full permission** to reread any textbook, rework any problems or work sheets, and rewrite any paper or assignment. You may also read ahead or behind in your text books as much as necessary to meet your time goals.

2) If you still don't meet your time goals, then you are to go back to your teachers and politely inform them that you are trying to study (for example) 15 minutes per night in their subject and **"could they please help you out with ideas about what to study?"** As we noted earlier, most teachers are *quite gracious* about helping students figure this out. This strategy is likely to be highly successful for you too!

3) The two suggestions above have solved the problem of how to fill up time for 99% of all our students. However, if they are not enough, you have our **complete permission** to go to your school library and check out 3 books related to your subjects and read those during your study time. Also, parents may know that the student needs to work on certain weaknesses and may **assign the student a particular task.** For example, parents may require their student to work on multiplication tables, spelling lists or independent reading.

THERE ARE NO EXCEPTIONS TO THIS RULE!

Parents: **do not** argue the "relative merits" of these rules with your children. The time-honored way for children to get you to change the rules is to get you into an argument about them. **If they can't get you into an argument, the rule is set and they know they have to do it.** The point is, your student must learn to use his/her mind in a disciplined way. This kind of reasonable structure is a way of loving your children.

In fact, if your student skips a night during the week we'd suggest you have them make up the time on Saturday morning.

Did You Negotiate Stopwatch Time?

You should have already negotiated the amount of stopwatch (on-task) study time your student will do each day this coming week and **written this number above the days of the week on his/her chart.** If you have not done this, do it now.

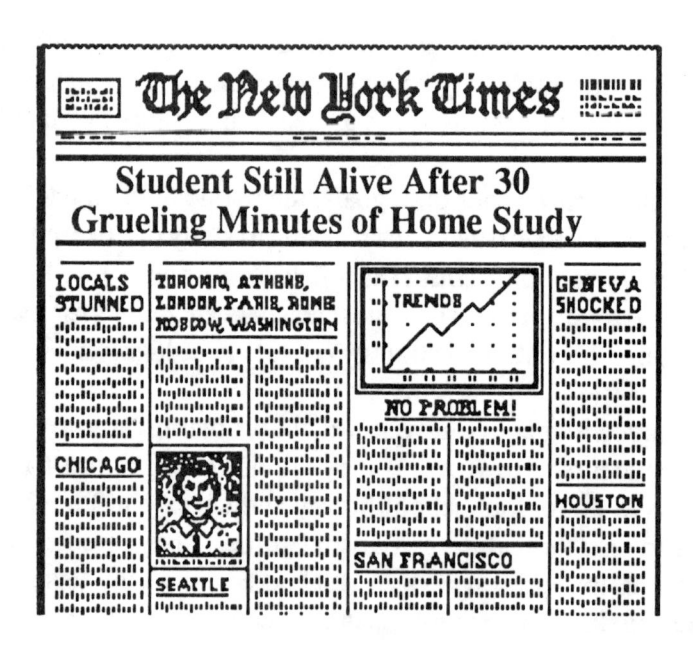

Last, but not least, comes the . . .

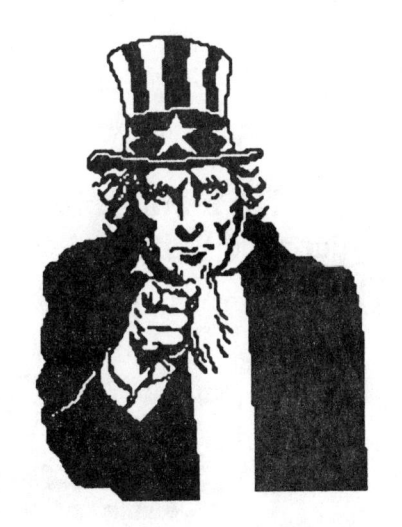

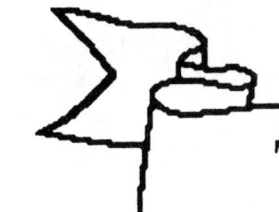

The Ten Commandments

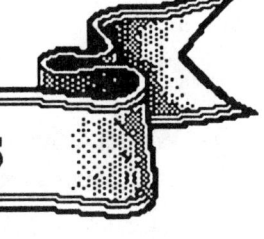

1) Begin at the **same time** every day.

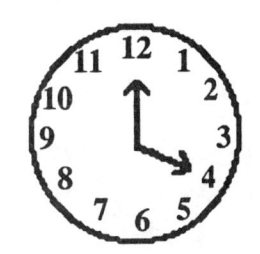

2) Pick a quiet place and sit in a **hard back chair** at a table or desk. DO NOT try to study on your bed (you know it makes you sleepy).

3) **Never try to study and watch TV at the same time.** The same applies to the radio and stereo. Why? These things are all serious business attempts to control your attention to make a profit.

4) Do not answer the telephone during study periods. **All calls should be taken by someone else** who will explain that you are studying and cannot be disturbed. You can call back later.

5) Before you start to study, **gather all the things you will need** before sitting down. Sharpen your pencils, have plenty of paper, get all your books and homework assignments and be ready to work.

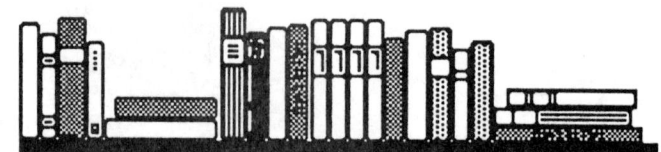

6) When you are ready with everything, **start your stopwatch.** Check your assignment sheet for the things you need to do. Remember, when your mind wanders you **must turn off your stopwatch!**

7) After you think you have memorized something, **spend more time overlearning** it. Under test pressure, it's often more difficult to remember things than you may have thought.

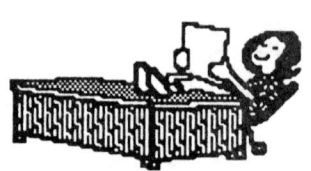

8) When you get an assignment that is not due to for several days (or even weeks), **you must work on it 15 minutes every night** starting from the first day you got the assignment *until it is done.*

			Calendar			
M 15	Tu 15	W 15	Th 15	F	S	S 15
M 15	Tu 15	W 15	Th Done	F	S	S
M	Tu	W	Th	F	S	S
M	Tu	W	Th	F	S	S

9) When you are done studying it is extremely important to **fill out your Study Plan immediately.** Have your parent initial it.

10) Now that you have taken care of your school obligations **go play with a clear conscience.** You've earned it!

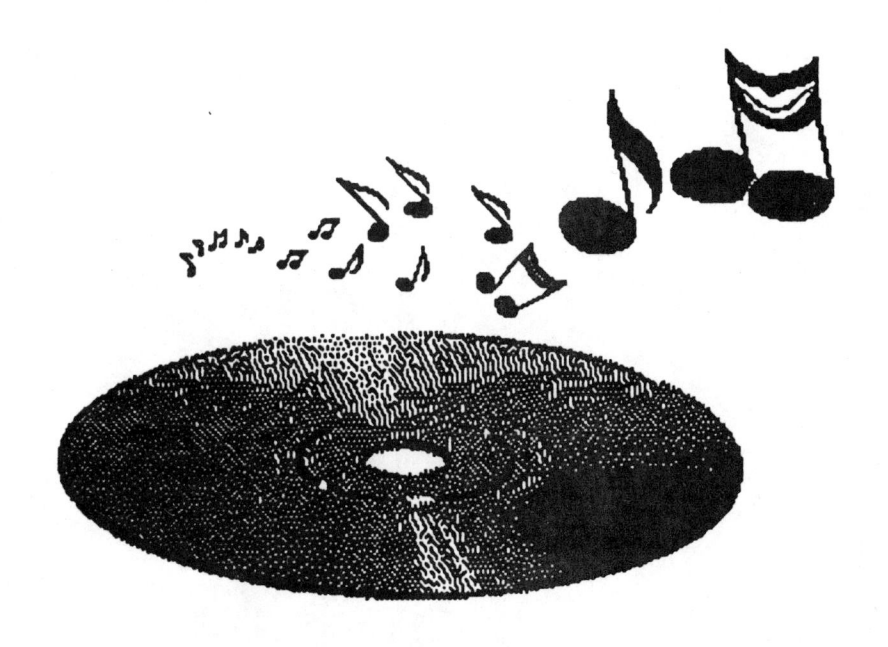

This is the end of Week One. *Do not* go to the next chapter, Week Two (or peek ahead!), until you have **studied for one week.** However, do be sure to **plan** the day of the week you will read Week Two.
Mark it on your home calendar.
See you next week!

Week 2

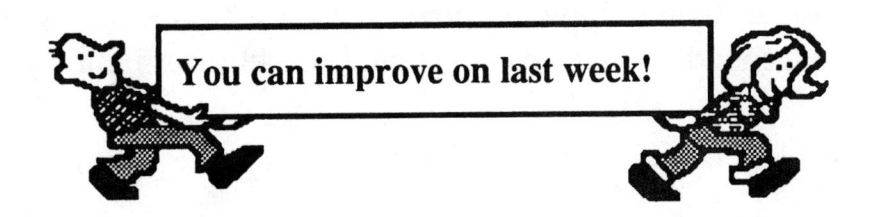

You can improve on last week!

The Case of the Missing Math Paper

Something was wrong here. Susan was an eighth grader who had started the Workshop not studying at all, but here we were, 7 weeks later and she was studying 90 minutes *every night*. The only problem was, she was still failing math and several other subjects. All "D's" and "F's." How on earth could that be?

Her parents vouched for the fact that she *really did study*. In fact, they were quite pleased with her in this regard. As it turned out, the problem actually, was with us. You see, this was the first workshop we had ever given and we were still fairly new at helping students. I had the nagging feeling we had overlooked something quite obvious for weeks now but couldn't quite put my finger on it. For the umpteenth time I ran down a mental checklist for failing students:

Was she on drugs? I really didn't think so.

Did she have a deep unconscious need to fail? Possible, but it didn't square with her working behavior.

Was she being abused? It hardly seemed likely. I had investigated child abuse earlier in my career for several years. Susan and her parents did not appear to be hiding things. They came on time and were open to making changes. Judging by the way they talked with each other, I felt they were a loving family.

Was it that she lacked sufficient intelligence? Well, she seemed about average to me in the speed at which she understood concepts. She didn't seem to have reading problems.

Did she have extreme problems relating to teacher authority? If she did, I didn't sense it in the way she related to me. She did want to know "why" sometimes when I asked her to do certain things, and sometimes she put up a mild protest. But really, she seemed pretty ordinary for an eighth grader in this respect. And she did do what she was asked to do: she was studying 90 minutes a night!

So, what was the problem? I returned to asking Susan questions about her week. Suddenly things started to fall into place as we talked about math (her most difficult subject).

Me: "Susan, you say you did your math this week, but didn't turn it in. How come?"
Susan (shrugs): "Well, I don't really know. I couldn't find it I guess."
Me (suspiciously): "Are you *sure* you really did it?
Susan: "Yeah, it's in here" (points to her PeeChee).
Me: "OK, so show it to me. The group and I will wait."

What happened next was unforgettable. Susan pulled out her PeeChee; it was **three inches thick!** The cover was badly ripped and torn. She had spent hours decorating it (it was beautiful) but it was old now, and in terrible shape. It looked like it was held together with glue, string, paper clips, saliva, several yards of colored tape, and the sheer force of her love for it.

As she carefully opened it on her lap, she balanced it on her knees *so that it wouldn't rip down the middle*. And then she started to thumb through the pages ever so carefully. I let her look for 5 minutes, which, in a group, probably felt like 50 minutes. She couldn't find it. I told her that I was good at finding things and would she please let me have a try.

I too handled this prized possession with the respect it deserved. I balanced it gently on *my* knees, and opened it with great ceremony.

You will have to pardon my naivety - I had never looked inside a junior high PeeChee before. I was so shocked by what I saw that I almost dropped it!

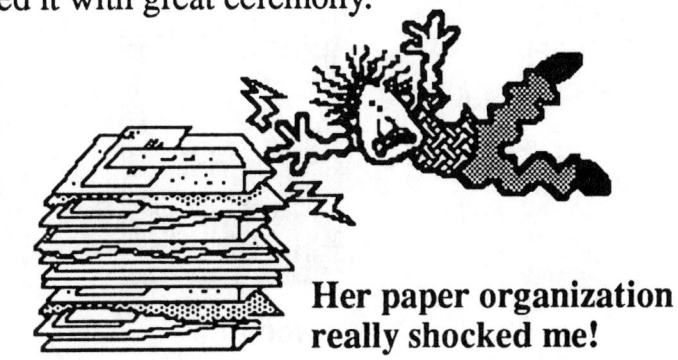

Her paper organization really shocked me!

I mean, there were papers in there that were **folded, smashed, wrinkled, smudged, ripped, crumpled, stapled, torn, taped, and clipped.** Furthermore, it was March and there was a *random wad of papers still there from early September* (to be fair about it, only the corners were starting to yellow with age).

Nothing was in order. The confusion was greatly enhanced by the fact that the papers were put in **upside down, sideways, backwards,** and occasionally, **right side up.**

Well, I couldn't find the elusive math paper either. So, to further diagnose the situation, I took out a clean sheet of paper and asked Susan to show me how she had filed it in her PeeChee. She took it and inserted it about 2/3 of the way in the back. We looked there for a couple minutes and eventually found the mystery paper - completely finished, with **nearly every problem done correctly, but unseen by educator eyes.**

Now, I do not believe in belittling people, and, if the truth be known, I dearly love children of all ages, colors, shapes, and sizes. So I was madly trying to think up a way to tactfully tell Susan she needed to make **a big change in her life.** What I managed was something like the following:

"Susan, I have just had a rather clear insight. I know you love your PeeChee, but I want you to retire it to an honored place in your room. I promise that your true individuality will not be stifled for the rest of your life."

(Turning to her mother) "Would you be willing to spend about $3.50 on a new three ring notebook today for this delightful child of yours who has a rather serious organizational problem?" (Actually, she was more than willing - *transcendent joy* might better describe her response.)

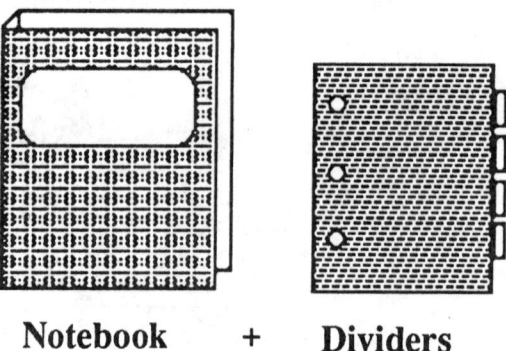

Notebook   +   Dividers   =   New Hope

26

I told Susan I would gladly give her stopwatch time to set up a three ring notebook with divider tabs for each subject that was **arranged in order by the date of the assignment.** In fact, I was happy to give her stopwatch time *every night* at the beginning of her study period to clean up her notebook on a daily basis.

She did it. The very next quarter, Susan got all "A" and "B" grades. She kept it up the whole next year, and got only an occasional "C" in hard subjects.

Even I didn't guess her true potential was this good.

Needless to say, some rather profound changes have also taken place in her self-concept. And her **true individuality has been greatly enhanced.**

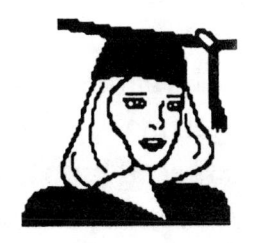

Do not assume that junior and senior high age students really know how to organize themselves if they have not been specifically taught. In fact, most do not.

> **Special Assignment:** If the student is not using a standard 3 ring notebook, buy him/her one as soon as possible and give the student stopwatch time to organize all papers in order by date in a separate section for each class. You will probably need to buy divider tabs for this purpose. **PeeChees and Trapper Keepers are NOT acceptable.** (Kids use trapper keepers like glorified PeeChees.)

We Are Mind Readers

About half of you did pretty well following directions and got most everything done last week. *Our compliments!* You are doing something exciting and we applaud your hard work. Your problems may not be serious and you are likely to do quite well working in this book over the next 7 weeks.

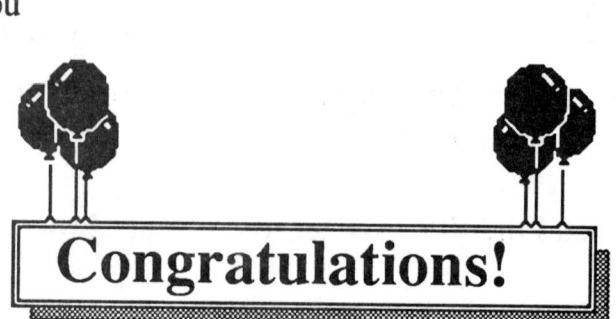

Congratulations!

The other half of you . . . Well . . . shall we say, you are the students we **most enjoy working** with because you stand to *grow the most* from this experience!

Parents: The second week is often the hardest week in this whole process. This is because some students will be "testing" you very hard about whether or not **they really have to study 5 days a week at home** (protests notwithstanding, this is not child abuse). If your student is not following through, we will give you help to more tightly structure the situation to make things work better. Remember, helping students "learn to learn" is a *high level parenting problem.* If you thought it would happen without your involvement, you probably wouldn't have bought this book. We simply **cannot allow our children to fail.** It takes love, and sometimes courage to face this kind of serious problem. But, left to themselves, failing students continue to fail: the rate of "spontaneous recovery" from a chronic problem like this is very, very low.

The (learned) ability to study effectively and follow through, is predictive of achievement in life.

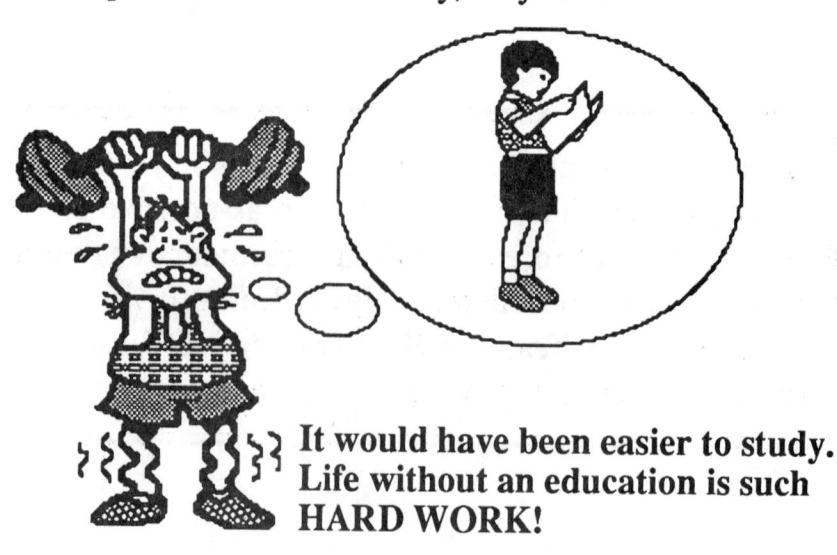

It would have been easier to study. Life without an education is such **HARD WORK!**

Some things can be compromised, others cannot. One of the priceless gifts you can give your teenage children before they leave home is the **uncompromising message** (with quiet, but firm structure) that regular, disciplined thinking (a) solves problems, (b) makes people feel good about themselves, and (c) improves the quality of life.

It is difficult work for all of us to give our children "hard love" but it's often worth it, and *we have all seen our children make real life changes that just don't happen any other way.* As one determined mother of a difficult student put it at the end of a Workshop:

"Thank you so much for:

1) Encouraging us to be assertive parents.
2) Helping us open doors that have rusted shut.
3) Giving each student honest and concerned attention that has helped each one take himself more seriously.
4) Somehow giving me the courage to "butt" into my son's life. This has let him know that I really care about him and his total growth - not just his stomach and a kiss goodnight.
5) Personally, I have been given a handle on certain attitudes I tolerate toward my own academic achievement.
6) This list could go on and on - so I'll sum it up by saying thank you again for giving my son and I a clearer view of our own potential."

Students: We just love kids. Really! All kinds of kids. And we think that whether you want to or not, you will be the next generation of adults to inherit the earth. In fact, the future of the whole planet (and our Social Security) will be in your hands. Furthermore, our generation never got around to fixing all (or even most) of the problems. There are **plenty** of "brain busters" left for you. In fact, it has gotten so complicated we don't even know where some of the problems are anymore.

Simple fact is, there are enough **really incredible problems** to go around for everybody. Which, in a way, can be good because *many problems are really opportunities in disguise.* Of course, most people don't know that, but if you do, and you develop your talent for solving problems, you will be in *very high demand someday.* Students can experience their own personal potential long before they enter the world of work. We want you to get "turned on" to the idea that it is exciting to **control your own life** with self-discipline and that solving problems with your mind is proof that you can make a positive difference in the world. We need you.

If you do not become part of the solution, you will become part of the problem.

Brief Reflection

I (Ross) will never forget a brief conversation I had years ago in high school with a bright, attractive girl who really wasn't working very hard. She said she didn't know who her future husband would be, or where he was, but she "certainly did hope he was out there studying hard and getting good grades."

She had to learn the hard way you can't leave that up to someone else.

Next, you will learn how to use the information you have gathered in the **Study Plan** and the **Assignment Sheet**.

How to Use the Study Plan and Assignment Sheet

The student has been collecting vital information for the past week. There are several basic uses to which you can both put this information. First of all, you must have **done it.** If you "blew" this critical function, you will find help in the next section, **Common Problems and Solutions.** If, however, you did a good job of recording things, you can begin to use this information positively like this:

1) The first thing you now have is a "baseline" that lets you know about how much the student actually studies. Save this sheet so that you have a basis to compare (and praise) your student in later weeks as he/she grows.

2) You may have already experienced more consistency in getting started with homework and in the amount of time studied. Parents: **be sure to let your student know you appreciate this.**

3) Some of you may realize you are "fighting less and enjoying it more." Give the student credit for this development.

4) Review the week using last week's **Study Plan.** Were the TV, radio, and stereo off? Was study done at a table or desk? Was it reasonably quiet in the house? (This is a parent responsibility.) Were **you** consistent about signing off the chart **every** night?

5) Now, look to see if the student is getting any "D" or "F" grades and has **little or no homework recorded for that subject** during the week. Do not get angry, this is common. Instead, **simply make a rule** that the student will ask the teacher what he/she needs to study and set a minimum of 10 minutes in that subject every night (or whatever parents think is reasonable, but don't overdo it). **Write this number** in the new study plan for the next week (see Kevin's **Study Plan** on the next page). Accept no excuses! If there is more than one poor grade, **don't try to tackle more than two** of them this week. Ask the student's advice about which subjects they can bring up the easiest and go with those.

This same method may be used in the case where the lowest grade the student is getting is a "C" or a "B," and is not studying enough for the class at home.

For example, Kevin needs to study 10 minutes every night in Math and Health so we mark it into his chart for the coming week under "subjects":

STUDY PLAN
Academic Skills Workshop
Daily Goals

Name: Kevin
Date: 10/30/88

Subjects:	30 W	30 Th	7 F	7 S	30 S	30 M	30 Tu	Week Total	Teacher Comments: Grade, Attitude, Work in?
English									
Math *10/night									(He had an F+ last week + only studied 5 minutes)
Social Studies									
Health *10/night									(He has a big assign due in 4 days)
Total Stopwatch Time									Weekly Average=____
Start/Finish									(Add total number of minutes for the week and divide by 5 days.)
Place You Studied									
Parent Initials									

6) We know from experience that the **Assignment Sheet** will have from 8 to 12 entries on it when it is being used properly. And it **Must be Used Properly!** If there are only about 3 or 4 entries the student probably did not do this correctly. Check the **dates carefully.** There should be entries yesterday and today.

7) Always look for small improvements and try to **balance the feedback you give your student with respect and positive expectations for their effort.** Realize you are only in the second week and it won't be perfect yet. That's OK, in fact, we expect it.

I'm proud of your effort this week!

Common Problems and Solutions

Problem 1: The student failed to record study time or to show the booklet to the parent. This is serious because it means the student is (a) in negative control of the situation, and (b) doing more poorly in school than is necessary.

The Solution: Actually, there are several. Often, students are waiting until they are "sure" they must study 5 days a week. When parents help their student solve the problem (and many of you will) it probably comes from the *tone of voice* and *body posture* you use when you really mean it. **When you really mean it (hard love), there are no valid excuses, and students often respond with improved behavior.** It is critically important that *you* be consistent.

If you have trouble conveying when you really mean it, you may want to read a short book called Back in Control, by Gregory Bodenhamer. Mr. Bodenhamer has developed practical techniques for parents to control behavior in delinquent teenagers. In our opinion, some of these techniques are strong enough to be harmful if misapplied. However, when used with compassion and good judgment, they can be effective when other means have not.

If this doesn't work, and you are a two parent family, you may consider having the other parent work with the child, or perhaps, have both of you work with the child together until the **child understands you will follow through.**

If that doesn't work, you may well wish to consider going to the school counselor for support and help, or to a family counselor. If there is a Workshop Leader for the **Academic Skills Workshop** (from which this book was developed) listed in appendix A, this is probably the best possible resource you can find.

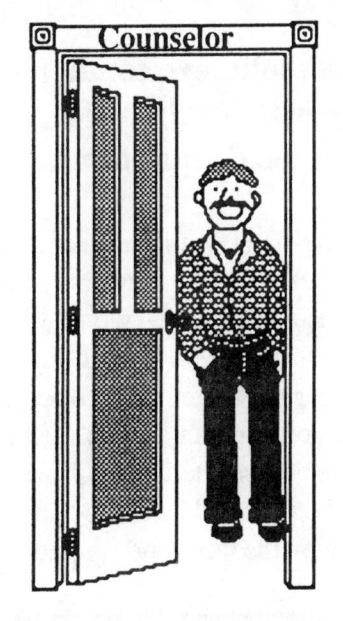

Welcome:

Office Hours: 9:00 a.m.
              5:00 p.m.

Evenings by appointment

The point is, if your child is calling the shots by refusing to study and complete a simple recording sheet, you have more than just a study skills problem.

Problem 2: Your child "forgets" to do homework and turn it in.

The Solution: Check the assignment sheet daily and ask probing questions about what is missing from it. This is best illustrated with a little digression.

Excuse Me, What DIDN'T You Say?

When I (Ross) worked as a therapy consultant in the prisons for men, and later women, I quickly learned there are two main kinds of lies; there are (1) direct lies, and (2) lies of omission.

When most people think of a lie, they generally think of direct lies (eg., "your ordinary bald-faced lie," like telling someone you were "at the Mall" when you were really at Jimmy's house).

Lies of omission happen when you know **darned well** that someone should know what you are doing and you don't tell them *because they didn't ask*, or they *didn't ask exactly the right question.* For example, **Question:** "Did you turn in your homework today dear?" **Answer:** "Yes, Mom." **Truth:** The student *did* turn in an overdue assignment in Social Studies today but *didn't turn in 3 math assignments earlier in the week.* This is the kind of lie we are concerned with, because they usually start **long before** direct lies are told.

There is a trick to confronting lies by omission that often works, even with "inmate experts" in prison. It requires that you:

1) **make solid eye contact**
2) **talk with a calm voice, and**
3) **ask specific questions.**

For example, I often got lies by omission when I would ask inmates general questions like "did you have any problems this week?" The answer was often a convincing "no," and only much later in the conversation (if at all) would I learn the inmate had been in a shouting match that ended just short of a physical fight, been disciplined by a guard, or had used drugs. I quickly learned to get **very concrete.** For example, I might **start** with a question like "have you used any drugs?" (they'd say "no") and then **follow it up** with, "does that include pot and alcohol?" Often the response would be, "well, maybe a little pot but I don't think that's a drug. You know, like *Heroin is a drug.*" At that point, the cards were on the table and we had our work cut out for us.

Likewise, parents can get good results by being direct with students who don't bring home assignments or turn them in. First, you must **get at the truth soon enough to help** (which, until your student is doing it responsibly, means **daily**). What usually has been happening is that the issue is so "hot" there is an unspoken agreement not to talk about it much for weeks at a time - other than a brief, but worried, "are you keeping up dear?" To which the student replies something like, "well, I'm sorta doin' OK mom," until the warning slips come home a few weeks later (and parents feel angry about being misled). This is not only destructive academically, but also **affects trust levels** at home. It must stop, and fair or not, the parent can (must) lead the way.

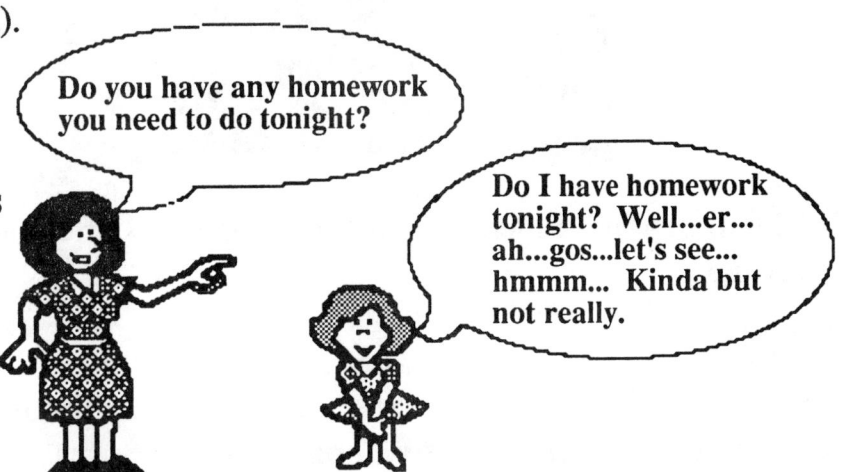

Do you have any homework you need to do tonight?

Do I have homework tonight? Well...er... ah...gos...let's see... hmmm... Kinda but not really.

The first step is to **absolutely insist the student fill out the assignment sheet on a daily basis.** At a minimum, parents should go over it with them at the same time they sign off their **Study Plan** each night. To be effective at this you must:

1) Make clear, **direct eye contact** (eyes are the "window to the soul").

2) Ask patiently **if anything is missing from the assignment sheet and if everything is turned in.** Do not hurry through this. Listen carefully with your ears, eyes, and intuition. Stay calm and follow up on any hesitation be it verbal or nonverbal. It works.

3) Whether the answer is yes or no, **ask if there is anything missing from each specific class,** "Is there any assignment not on this **Assignment Sheet** from Math? English? Social Studies? Science? Health?" and etc.

4) Have your student **write down any "forgotten" assignments** he/she "remembers" on the assignment sheet right away. If they are due the next day, they must complete them immediately, even if they have already put in "all their study time."

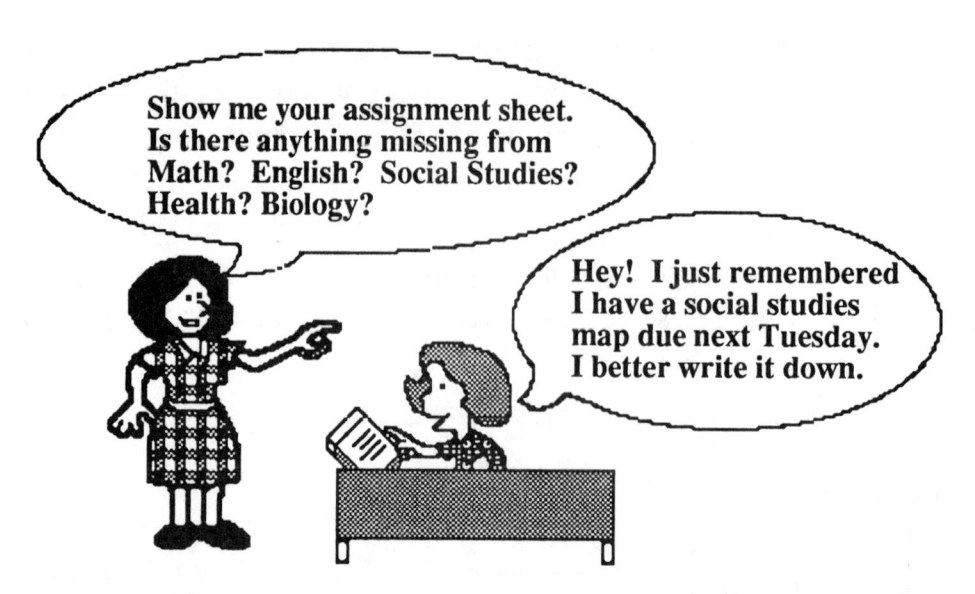

> Show me your assignment sheet. Is there anything missing from Math? English? Social Studies? Health? Biology?

> Hey! I just remembered I have a social studies map due next Tuesday. I better write it down.

Problem 3: The student procrastinates getting started on homework nearly every day.

The Solution: Set a time to get started by, for example, 7:00 p.m. (this the latest we typically allow students to start, otherwise they become too tired to think well). Give the student **exactly 15 minutes "grace"** past this time to be seated in a hard back chair at a table or desk and studying. If the student is not actively working on homework at **7:15 p.m. and ONE SECOND,** add 20 minutes to the expected study time for the night. Don't argue the merits of this with your student. Both of you know it was set up in advance and it's fair. This is a good solution that **really works.**

Problem 4: The student has study goals that are "too low."

Solution: Relax! You are in this for the "long haul." As long as the student is following through with studying 5 days a week, this is the easiest problem to solve over the long run. In the beginning, it is very important **not to overload students with time expectations.** It is good enough that they work 5 days a week and begin to develop regular study habits. In general, we think the following stopwatch times are where students should be in 8 weeks:

Grades 4-6, 30-45 **on-task** minutes/night, 4 nights per week.
Grades 7-9, 45-75 **on-task** minutes/night, 5 nights per week.
Grades 10-12, 60-90 **on-task** minutes/night, 5 nights per week.

At this second week, students are at very different levels of study. Mostly it has to do with how much they studied before starting this system. If your student was a "dedicated nonstudier" and started out with 20 minutes per night, you are being very successful at this point! If your student was already studying before starting this book, and was mature enough to handle 45-60 minutes at the start, you should really let them know you appreciate it! In either case you can use judgment about adding 5-10 minutes per night each week until you reach a respectable maintenance level within the guidelines above.

As you come close to the optimal amount of study time for your student, both of you need to "feel your way to the balancing point." If you go past it (require too much time), the entire system will collapse.

There is no hurry, study skills are for a lifetime. Good things are happening now and as long as you follow the guidelines in this book, they will get easier and grow stronger.

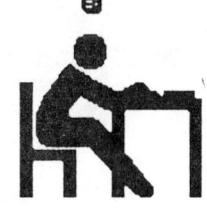

On the next page you will find The Checklist. Parents and students are to do this together.

The Checklist

(Parent and Student do together)

Special Focus: Recording in Chart

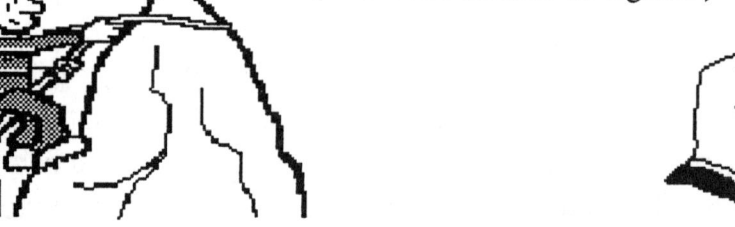

Mark the following **yes** or **no** as was true of your week:

___ The student **used the stopwatch and recorded accurate times at each study period.**

___ The student made his/her contracted study goal for the week or worked on Saturday morning until the contracted study time was made up. (Note: It is a parent responsibility to ask about this and to enforce it if necessary).

___ If the student has assignments that are not due immediately, he/she worked on them for at least 15 minutes each night or until they were done.

___ The student took the Study Plan to all teachers for comments once during the week. Low grades were compared with minutes spent on that subject during the past week and any needed time increases for next week were made and written into the Study Plan.

___ The student recorded every assignment, test, and quiz in the Assignment Sheet.

___ The student turned in every assignment this week.

___ The student took the Study Plan to his/her parent for their initials after every study period.

These are the minimum requirements you will rate every week until the end of the book.

Now, Put These Ideas to Work

We haven't finished dealing with everything that can come up but you have many practical ideas to try at this point. To summarize, these are:

1) **Negotiate the amount of study time** and enter it on a new **Study Plan** (a new Study Plan and Assignment Sheet are at the end of this chapter). Put the new Assignment Sheet and Study Plan at the *front of the student's regular school notebook* and be sure all school subjects are listed on the new Study Plan. Have your student **record his/her study time every day.** Parent's initial the Study Plan. **Don't skip the initials!** If your student didn't bring the Study Plan to you to initial last week, ask to see it each night.

2) If your student procrastinates, set a time to begin and allow 15 minutes and ONE SECOND leeway, then **assign an extra 20 minutes of homework**.

3) See that your student has a **quiet place to study** at a table or a desk. No TV, no radio, no stereo, no phone calls during study time.

4) The student **must use the stopwatch correctly.** NO EXCEPTIONS.

5) Check and **initial the assignment sheet daily** if your student is having trouble turning in assignments. If your child loses the assignment sheet or the study plan, begin a new one the same day. NO EXCEPTIONS!

6) Once a week, make sure your student gets a **teacher signature** for each academic class.

7) This can be a tough week! If you need extra support, **make an appointment** to talk with a teacher, counselor, or principal.

THERE IS NO SUCH THING AS NOT HAVING HOMEWORK! The only students who say this are underachieving. Remember, the student can (a) study ahead or behind and/or rework assignments, (b) ask teachers for help and/or extra credit to fill up homework time, and (c) check out three books related to his/her subjects from the library to read during study time.

Parents may also know that the student needs to work on certain weaknesses and may assign the student a particular task. For example, parents may require their student to work on math facts, spelling lists, or independent reading.

Go over Your Checklist

Now, return to your Checklist on page 38 and make a plan with your student to correct any of the items that were answered "no." **Do it Now**

If you didn't have any "no's" you are doing unusually well, it doesn't happen very often in the second week. Finally, you have already negotiated the amount of study time the student will study and the student should have **written it into the new Study Plan** for the coming week. If for any reason this hasn't been done, do it now.

You are now set.

If either of you are even a little concerned that you may have a misunderstanding about your exact agreement, you may write your plan below.

_____

_____

_____

_____

_____

STOP

This is the end of Week Two. On the next two pages are a new **Study Plan** and **Assignment Sheet.** You may use these this week but *do not* go to the next chapter, Week Three, until you have studied for one week. However, do be sure to **plan** the day of the week you will read Week Three and mark it on your home calendar.
See you next week!

Study Plan
Academic Skills Workshop

Name: _____
Date: _____

Daily Goals

Subjects:						Week Total	Teacher Comments: Grade/Attitude/All Work Turned In?

Total Stopwatch Time For All Subjects:

When Did You Start?
When Did You Finish?

Place You Studied:

Parent's Initials:

WEEKLY AVERAGE = _____ Minutes/Day
(Add total number of minutes for the week and divide by 5 days.)

COPYRIGHT © January 1, 1988 by Counseling and Workshop Professionals
Unauthorized Reproductions Are Illegal and may be Punishable by Large Fines.
Students who have individually purchased this book may make copies for their own personal use. Copies may not be made for friends. School Districts are **Expressly Forbidden** to replicate these materials. A special discount is available to schools. Call (503) 588-1010 for ordering information.

Assignment Sheet

Write down the exact assignment before leaving class

Class	Assignment	Date Given	Date Due	Date Turned In	Parent Initials

Week 3

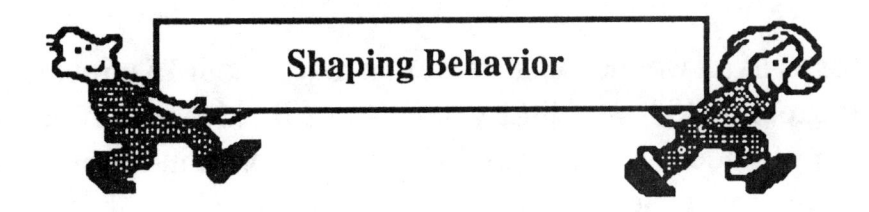

Shaping Behavior

On the Care and Training of Pigeons
(How To Shape Positive Behavior)

With literary license in hand we tell you the following story. It is in based on an actual experience. However, the "details" have, well . . ., shall we say, "matured" with many years of retelling (some irrational skeptics might accuse us of outright fabrication).

He Got Our Attention . . .

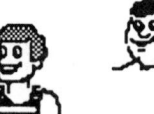

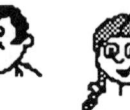

Many years ago, when I (Ross) was a college sophomore, I signed up for a course in Experimental Psychology. One day, without warning, I came to class to find the other 29 students buzzing in the room around 15 rather nervous looking pigeons in cages. There were also 15 tall, square cardboard boxes, scissors, rolls of tape, and little containers of pigeon food. It figured to be a different kind of day.

The professor let us all wonder what he was up to for about 15 minutes and then he entered the room. With very little ceremony he divided us up into pairs and gave each pair of students a pigeon and a red dot one inch in diameter. He told us all to paste the dot on the inside of the cardboard box about "beak high," put our pigeon in the box, and train them to peck the dot. He gave us 30 minutes.

The first thing that happened was that about 5 or 6 of the birds escaped and started flapping around the room and dropping the "little gifts" for which pigeons have attained lasting fame.

Mother told me there would be days like this.

Those of us who actually got our bird in the box faced a novel set of problems. Mostly, the birds just flapped their wings, shuffled their feet, and cocked their heads nervously. We weren't at all sure how to proceed.

Many different approaches were tried:

Some of us tried to "make friends" by putting bird seed in our hands and lowering it down to the pigeons. Mostly they acted scared and flapped away as best they could.

Others tried dropping little bits of bird seed on the floor of the box. The birds ate it, but it didn't do much to train them to peck the dot.

Some students tried tapping on the side of the box when the birds went the wrong way and expressed verbal disapproval (the least of which were names like "bird brain").

After several unrewarding approaches, some otherwise intelligent college students were "sweet talking" their birds and pleading with them to peck the dot because they "didn't want to fail the experiment did they?"

Finally, the less sympathetic among us simply reached down, grabbed the birds by the neck, and tapped their beak on the dot by way of demonstration. Still, evidence of lasting comprehension was sadly lacking.

When it was over, we generally held pretty dim views about both pigeon training and intelligence.

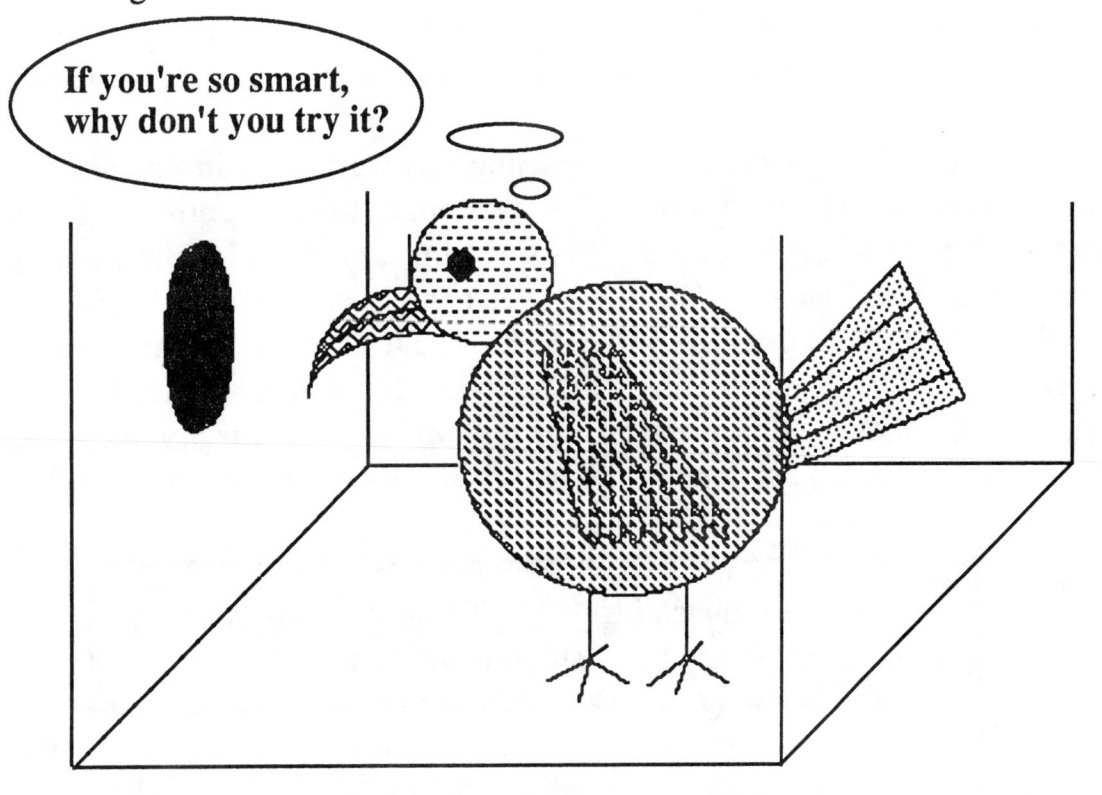

Then The Professor Showed Us How To Do It . . .

He took one of the cardboard boxes and cut a little hole near the bottom. This was for a food tray that he made so he could choose when to feed the bird.

Next he "borrowed" one of our birds and put it in the box. He waited a minute for the bird to calm down. Then, when the bird moved *just a toenail of a step toward the dot by accident,* he presented the food tray (through the hole he had cut in the box) and let the bird eat a few pecks. Then he removed the food tray. While he was doing this he explained that none of the birds had eaten that day because "it always helps to work with a motivated pigeon."

He continued to wait for the bird to *make a little bit more* of a move toward the dot before offering food. Soon the bird was quickly moving toward the dot and standing in front of it. Next, he waited until the bird made a random movement of its head toward the dot and then he fed it again. Shortly thereafter the bird brushed the dot with his beak and soon it was pecking the dot. The whole process took less than 10 minutes in the hands of this professor who was skilled at *shaping behavior.*

Behavior Shaping

Of course, shaping behavior in human beings is infinitely more complicated and challenging than pigeons! We tell you this story to help make a few points.

First, you probably noticed that the most important difference in whether or not the pigeon learned to do something new, was **not in the motivation or desires of the trainer** (we all *wanted* our bird to peck the dot), it was in how the pigeon trainer (professor) *set up a situation* in which the pigeon *could not fail.* If you really understand all this, you will have noticed that the professor's behavior was **quite different** from the students' behavior. If the students wanted to train their pigeon, they would have to *change their approach to the problem.* Here we come to a truth most parents have experienced but tend to forget easily:

> **If we want our children's behavior to change, we frequently must change our own first.**

Simply put, if what you have been doing isn't working, you use your problem solving skills to *change your approach*. That means you will be doing something different (your behavior has changed).

Secondly, behavior shaping requires *great patience* and the *ability to notice small improvement*. There is a tremendous difference, for example, between the step-by-step commitment to solving little problems on a daily basis as in this book, and an angry "how could you flunk math! You should *want* to study." (There is no more sure way to "hook" your student's rebelliousness than to talk with them angrily like this. And, not to put too fine a point on it, but, honestly, did you, yourself, *want* to study when you were in school?)

Thirdly, when adaptive behavior is *consistently* shaped by parents over long periods of time (years) there is a very high probability that the student will *internalize as a self-rule what was once an external rule.* This always takes time. But, parents who care enough about their student's achievement to **make rational rules, patiently apply them every day, and always look for positive ways to highlight small steps forward,** will set the stage for their student to develop a great gift: self-discipline and confidence.

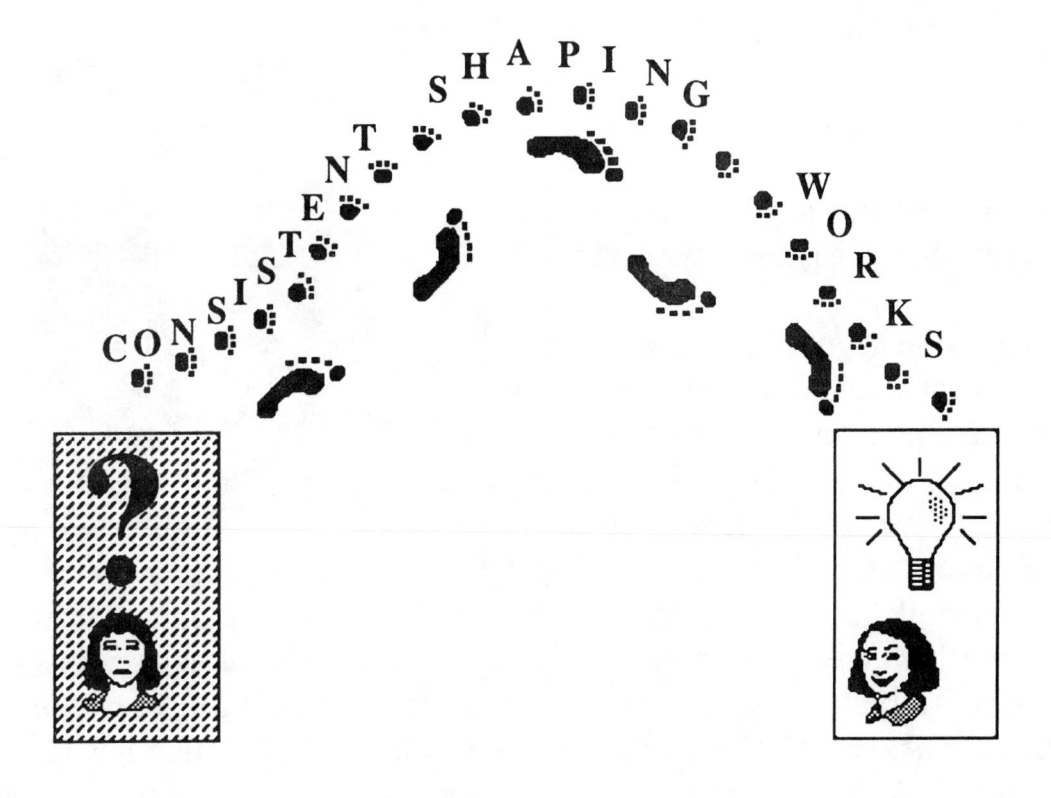

Common Problems and Solutions

Problem 1: The student is still not **reliably** bringing work home and turning it in on time.

The Solution: It's time to move up to the next level of intervention if your student has not responded by now. You must be prepared to consistently follow through for several months. The pattern of not bringing work home or turning it in has it's basis in (a) denial (the student does not recognize there is a serious problem) and (b) lies by omission (the student knows perfectly well you'd want to know but doesn't tell you). The typical parent response to both of these things is anger. Unfortunately, that will probably lead to a "hot" argument in which both parent and student lose (lose-lose pattern), or one in which the student "wins" and the parent loses because the parent gets frustrated and gives up (win-lose pattern). It is *very rare* for parents to walk away from a "hot" argument with a student feeling good, like they "won."

However, we certainly are not advocating that you simply let your student fail, or do poorly, and not use your own personal power to try to effect genuine change. But this needs to be set up so that you both ultimately win (win-win pattern). We will grant you that in the beginning your student may not experience studying as "winning," but of course it is.

<u>Advice On This Problem</u>

Do not: yell, blame, plead, use sarcasm, say negative things, pay money, *or* give up.

Do refuse to argue, then: look over the assignment sheet, make direct eye contact, and take your time to ask *specific* questions about *each* subject. Follow-up on any hesitation, and have your student **write down** missing work immediately. If your student says he/she is trying but just *can't remember* to bring work home from school, buy them an inexpensive digital wrist watch and help them *set the alarm for one minute after school is out* as a reminder. If the issue is turning work in, pick a specific class and *set the alarm for one minute after the class begins* to remind them to turn work in. Follow through the next day to make sure this happened. **Also, be sure the student's notebook is well organized.**

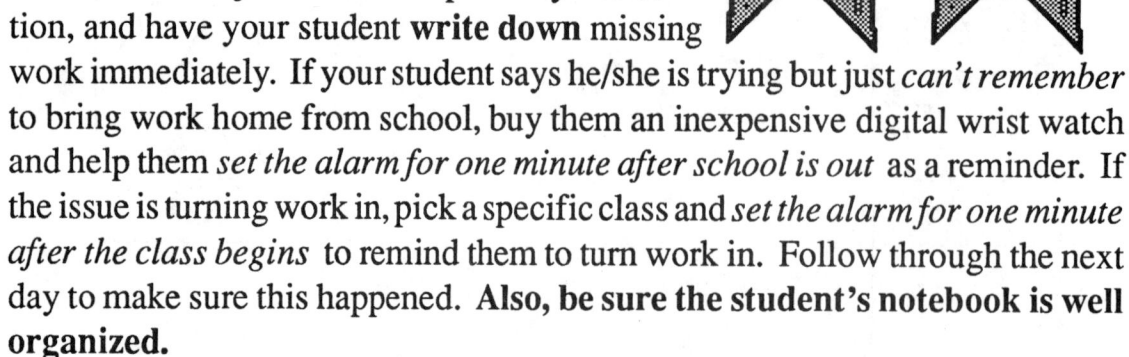

If you *find yourself tempted to argue,* try using two rule-based words "discovered" by Gregory Bodenhamer - **"nevertheless"** and **"regardless."** For example, the student might say something like, "hardly anybody in class turns this stuff in - the teacher doesn't even look at it!" Rather than "argue the merits of the case" (as framed up by the student), the parent consistently responds with conviction and patience, **"Nevertheless,** finish your homework and turn it in." After you have made your point, *leave the room* with the expectation set that your student will finish the work.

Problem 2: The student complains of being "bored" in class.

The Solution: First, understand that boredom in school is a result of (1) inattentiveness, (2) lack of interest or, *most commonly*, (3) lack of comprehension. When your student complains of boredom, it often means that he/she **is not trying very hard, or has given up.** (Parents - this *may also* be a sign the curriculum is too easy or difficult for your child and you need to have a school conference to find out.) In classes in which the student is "bored" the best solution we know of is to *require the student to ask at least two questions per day in class* and record that they did it on the Study Plan (use the numbers "1" and "2" for recording).

This works because:

1) Classes are about 45 to 50 minutes long.

2) It takes active listening to think up a question (it can take 5-10 minutes to think up a good question).

3) When students ask a question they are "center stage" for a brief time. This usually means the student experiences a mild, but stimulating *physical reaction* to being noticed. The aftereffects of this can last 5-10 minutes.

4) Thus, when students ask about two questions per period, they are more involved mentally and physically in the class. It often becomes more interesting. At a minimum, attention will be better focused and comprehension improves.

Problem 3: The student complains none of their friends has to study like this.

First, a reflection: Unfortunately, this is true. The great majority of students *are* disorganized and *do* have poor study habits and attitudes. Consider this:

a) When I (Ross) did my doctoral study to help junior high students who were doing poorly in public school, I made it a requirement that in order to receive help, students had to have at least one "D" or "F" in the first quarter. **I was shocked to find that 45% of all 7th and 8th graders qualified for my study!**

b) I often ask junior high counselors what percentage of students have *at least some problem turning assignments in on time.* I usually hear an estimate between 60 and 90%. Students in academic distress often guess 99% (!)

c) When you combine this with the the fact that 1 out of 4 students in junior high will not graduate from high school, you begin to understand the scope and seriousness of the problem.

So, indeed, *it is true* that many of your student's friends *do not study and organize themselves* very well. But is that what you want for your child? Of course not.

The Solution: Beyond a bemused tolerance for nonsense, don't argue the "merits" of this case with your "Philadelphia Lawyer." The **only** loving and appropriate response that helps your child in the long run, is, "nevertheless...." Then close the discussion.

> But the Supreme Court ruled in section 5, article b of the Uniform Student Code that no student shall be required to study and turn in work unless it can be shown "beyond a reasonable doubt" that it is absolutely necessary

> Nevertheless, Do Your Homework.

On the next page comes the Checklist.

The Checklist

(Parent and Student do together)

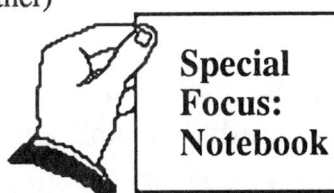

Special Focus: Notebook

Mark the following **yes** or **no** as was true of your week:

___ The student used the stopwatch and recorded accurate times at each study period.

___ The student is now using **a standard 3 ring notebook with divider tabs. All sections are arranged in logical order by subject and date.** (This is so important, it will be the special focus next week too.)

___ The student made his/her contracted study time or worked Saturday morning until the contracted time was made up. (Note: It is a parent responsibility to ask about this and to enforce it if necessary.)

___ If the student has assignments that are not due immediately, he/she worked on them for at least 15 minutes each night or until they were done.

___ The student took the Study Plan to all teachers for comments once during the week.

___ The student recorded every assignment, test, and quiz in the Assignment Sheet. Low grades were compared with minutes spent on that subject during the past week and any needed time increases for next week were made and written into the Study Plan.

___ The student turned in every assignment this week.

___ The student took the Study Plan to his/her parent for their initials after every study period.

These are the minimum requirements you will rate every week until the end of the book. Next use the **Study Skills Summary**.

Study Skill Summary

Parent and Student do Together

1) **Negotiate the amount of study time** and enter it on a new **Study Plan** (a new Study Plan and Assignment Sheet are at the end of this chapter). Put the new Assignment Sheet and Study Plan at the *front of the student's regular school notebook* and be sure all school subjects are listed on the new Study Plan. Have your student **record his/her study time every day.** Parent's initial the Study Plan. **Don't skip the initials!** If your student didn't bring the Study Plan to you to initial last week, ask to see it each night.

2) If your student procrastinates, set a time to begin and allow 15 minutes and ONE SECOND leeway, then **assign an extra 20 minutes of homework**.

3) See that your student has a **quiet place to study** at a table or a desk. No TV, no radio, no stereo, no phone calls during study time.

4) The student **must use the stopwatch correctly.** NO EXCEPTIONS.

5) Check and **initial the assignment sheet daily** if your student is having trouble turning in assignments. If your child loses the assignment sheet or the study plan, begin a new one the same day. NO EXCEPTIONS!

6) Once a week, make sure your student gets a **teacher signature** for each academic class.

7) This can be a tough week too! If you need extra support, **make an appointment** to talk with a teacher, counselor, or principal.

THERE IS NO SUCH THING AS NOT HAVING HOMEWORK! The only students who say this are underachieving. Remember, the student can (a) study ahead or behind and/or rework assignments, (b) ask teachers for help and/or extra credit to fill up homework time, and (c) check out three books related to his/her subjects from the library to read during study time.

Parents may also know that the student needs to work on certain weaknesses and may assign the student a particular task. For example, parents may require their student to work on math facts, vocabulary, spelling lists, or independent reading.

Go over Your Checklist

Now, return to your Checklist on page 51 and make a plan with your student to correct any of the questions that were answered "no." **Do it now**

You should have already negotiated the amount of study time the student will study and the student should have **written it into the Study Plan.** If for any reason this hasn't been done, do it now.

You are now set for the coming week.

If either of you are even a little concerned that you may have a misunderstanding about your exact agreement, you may write your plan below.

_____

_____

_____

_____

STOP

This is the end of Week Three. On the next two pages are a new **Study Plan** and **Assignment Sheet.** You may use these this week but *do not* go to the next chapter, Week Four, until you have studied for one week. However, do be sure to **plan** the day of the week you will read Week Four and mark it on your home calendar.
See you next week!

Study Plan
Academic Skills Workshop

Name: _____

Date: _____

Daily Goals

Subjects:										Week Total	Teacher Comments: Grade/Attitude/All Work Turned In?

Total Stopwatch Time For All Subjects:						WEEKLY AVERAGE = _____ Minutes/Day
When Did You Start?						(Add total number of minutes for the week and divide by 5 days.)
When Did You Finish?						
Place You Studied:						
Parent's Initials:						

COPYRIGHT © January 1, 1988 by Counseling and Workshop Professionals
Unauthorized Reproductions Are Illegal and may be Punishable by Large Fines.
Students who have individually purchased this book may make copies for their own personal use. Copies may not be made for friends. School Districts are **Expressly Forbidden** to replicate these materials. A special discount is available to schools. Call (503) 588-1010 for ordering information.

Assignment Sheet

Write down the exact assignment before leaving class

Class	Assignment	Date Given	Date Due	Date Turned In	Parent Initials

Week 4

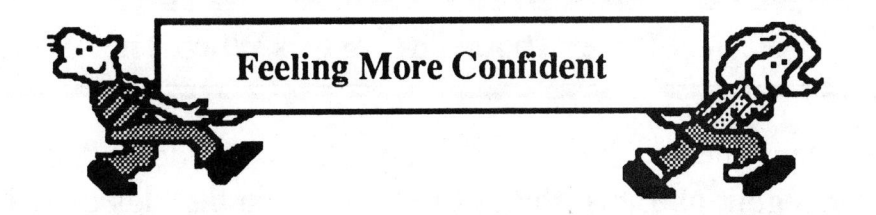

Feeling More Confident

Feeling More Confident

One of the great side-effects of solid study habits is the self-confidence that comes with it. By now, at the fourth week, there are *undoubtedly some students who are feeling better about themselves.* Many students have reached 40 to 60 minutes per night average and are more mature about how they handle school. They have more to do, but they are growing.

In fact, many students begin to experience a *rise in self-esteem.* Some students are unable to verbalize it, but *perceptive parents can see it* in their children. We have even seen school behavior problems like fighting simply stop. Once the *effort to improve* begins in earnest, many former failing students no longer identify easily with the kids who are acting-out and who don't try in school. All on their own, working students often find a new peer group that more closely matches their own feelings about themselves.

There is a simple reason for this:

It's magic!

People Feel Better About Themselves When They Work

What has happened is that nearly every child who doesn't do homework **experiences guilt about it** (this is true even when the kids deny it - that's a defense mechanism). You see, it is not just the feeling of productivity that doing work gives to students, it's also the *absence of guilt* that allows a more healthy sense of self-esteem to develop.

Small wonder that children respond so quickly.

There is no change that takes place in counseling that gives us more sheer pleasure than looking into the relaxed, yet alert faces of students who finally know the truth about themselves: **they can do it.**

Boy, do I feel good!

The next section is about **Parent Modeling.**

57

Parent Modeling

Parents: We need to talk with you quite directly this week because we'd like for you to think about what you *model* about learning and self-discipline for your students. That is, the things your children learn by your example, not your words. Allow us to paint a brief picture of two "middle class" homes.

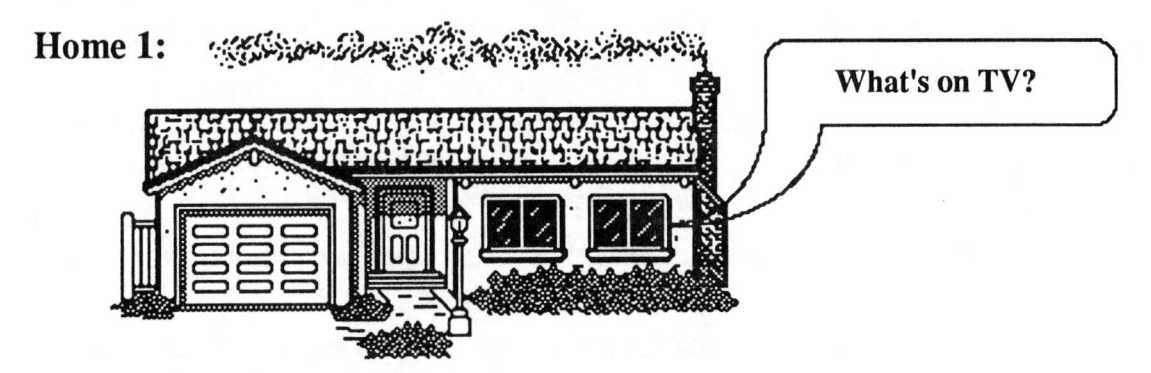

Home 1:

What's on TV?

* The parents watch TV *most every night.*
* They *rarely read* on their own for pleasure or information. It's been more than a year since either read a novel. On a good day, the kids see them read the newspaper.
* *Neither parent exercises* and both are overweight. One of them smokes.
* When the father comes home from work, he *plops in his chair* in front of the TV. More often than not, he has a drink.
* For outside entertainment they usually go to *movies or they bowl.*
* They really have *no intellectual interests* outside the home.
* They are *not involved* in their child's school parent group.
* Until a crisis hits, they *really don't know* much about what their child is learning in school. They haven't looked at the textbooks their student brings home.

In short, these parents model *little intellectual curiosity* for their children. They are nice enough people, but they *act as if learning for themselves is not important,* although they wouldn't say that to their children.

Home 2:

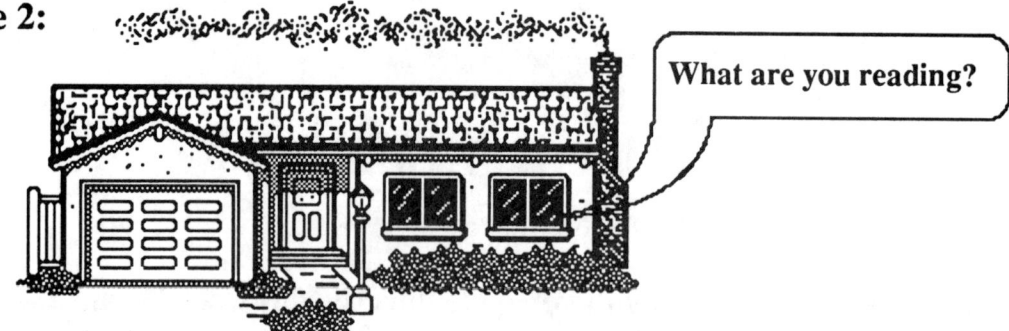

What are you reading?

* Both parents *read nearly every day*. It might be newspapers, newsletters, magazines, novels, vocational/technical books - anything. They share interesting tidbits with family members.
* TV is *off limits* most nights. When they watch, it's something special.
* They realize that good health is a precious gift. While they are not perfect about it, they *take care of their own bodies*. They gave up smoking or never started in the first place.
* When they come home, they *try to greet family members in a positive, interested way*, even when tired.
* For outside entertainment, the parents look forward to an evening at a local live theater as a treat and *like to take their children*. They may also go for recreation to see dance or ballet, hear concerts, visit libraries and museums, listen to lectures, and take field trips to just about anywhere.
* Both parents have *intellectual interests and hobbies* they pursue on their own.
* They care passionately about their child's education and *show it* by going to every conference and school function possible. They are active members of the school parent group.
* They *go over their child's school work* with supportive interest on a regular basis. They know what their child is learning in school and actively support it at home.

In short, these parents are intellectually alive and model the *effort, interest* and *persistence* that is characteristic of **life-long learners.**

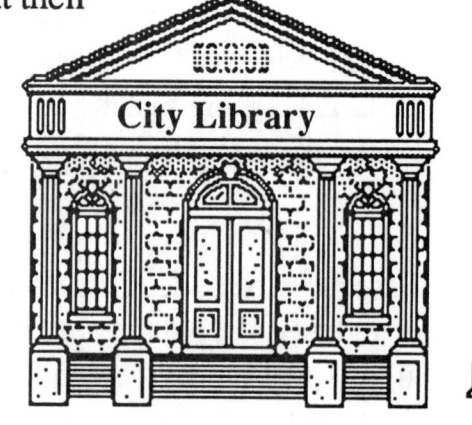

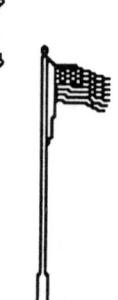

In Which Home Are You Mostly Likely To Find a "Turned On" Student?

Obviously in the second one. The modeling we do, both positive and negative, has a powerful influence on our children. It's *much stronger than the good advice we give.*

Additionally, parents *must have taken care of the basic problems* related to family stability for children to learn. Except for the few cases in which students withdraw from the family to do long hours of school work as a way to avoid conflict, it is *nearly impossible for children to learn at their potential* when families have serious problems. An *incomplete list* includes problems like alcoholism and drug use; physical, emotional, or sexual abuse; swearing and sarcasm; frequent angry arguing between parents; spouse battering or simply the fear of violence. Under circumstances like these, demanding full academic performance from children is irrational, self-defeating, and hypocritical. The child's first priority must be *how to survive* an irrational situation.

For those parents who see *even one* family problem in this list, you must find the courage to address the core problem first. Stability allows potential to unfold: we have seen dramatic academic progress in the teenage children of alcoholics when their parent/s go into treatment and begin recovery. This is the ideal time for us to work our system with these students.

A Modeling Story

Mr. "Herrera" was a working single father raising two boys. He was facing a difficult situation; his first grade son was not learning to read, even after two years of kindergarten. As commonly happens, when he fell further and further behind his peers, he began to act-out by getting into lots of fights. He was also becoming passively defiant in class by refusing to do work. He was a very discouraged child who could only "say it" by acting-out.

Mr. Herrera came from a migrant background. As a result, he himself had never learned how to read, and he felt that to survive as a child he had had to learn to fight. It was clear that his son, who was not under the same kind of environmental stress, was modeling after his father. Once the school understood the problem, many things were done which included setting up a school plan to stop the fighting, and a vision problem was identified which was corrected with glasses.

However, it still remained that this little boy was very far behind and was not enthused about school. This is where Mr Herrera, at age 40, accepted the challenge to step forward and lead the way for his son by *learning to read himself*. As you can imagine, he had to overcome internal obstacles himself to believe he could do it. At his age, he had accepted his reading inability as a fact of life that wasn't going to change. However, he *immediately understood* the logic of modeling, and there was *nothing more important to him* than that his boys should learn to read and receive the good education he had not.

The school arranged for a volunteer reading tutor to meet with him in his home. Mr. Herrera didn't say much about what he was doing to his boys. In fact, they were puzzled about why this strange person was in the house. After the second session, the tutor told me the boys could no longer contain their curiosity and approached the table and asked their dad what he was doing. Mr. Herrera looked up with a broad smile and said, "I'M LEARNING TO READ."

The result has been most gratifying. A year later, Mr. Herrera had made great progress. And the school began sending written notes to him about his son's progress. They said his son was *learning to read,* showing *interest in school,* and *no longer having serious behavior problems.*

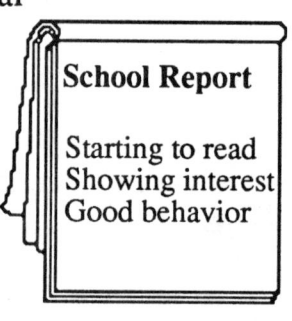

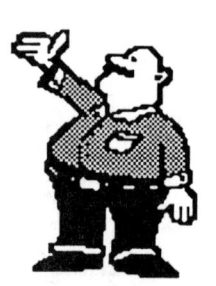

School Report

Starting to read
Showing interest
Good behavior

Next turn to the next section entitled **Improve Your Memory.** This begins a new emphasis in the book. We assume that if you have progressed this far that the student is recording stopwatch times faithfully on the **Study Plan,** you are getting feedback from teachers once a week, and that both you and your student think this method is reasonable and not some new form of child abuse. We will still offer behavior management tips, but now we also want to teach you skills that are more academic in nature.

IMPROVE YOUR MEMORY

Very few students know how to make really good use of their own capacity for memory. Like most things in life, the job is much easier, and the results more gratifying, when you use a disciplined method. The ability to remember well in school can be broken into two major parts (1) Overlearning, and (2) Mnemonic Devices.

Overlearning (Basic Facts)

1) You will remember best when you first **tell yourself to remember.** This is commonly overlooked: most students simply pick up a book and start reading. It is critical that you make a *commitment to yourself* in order to remember information after a few days have passed.

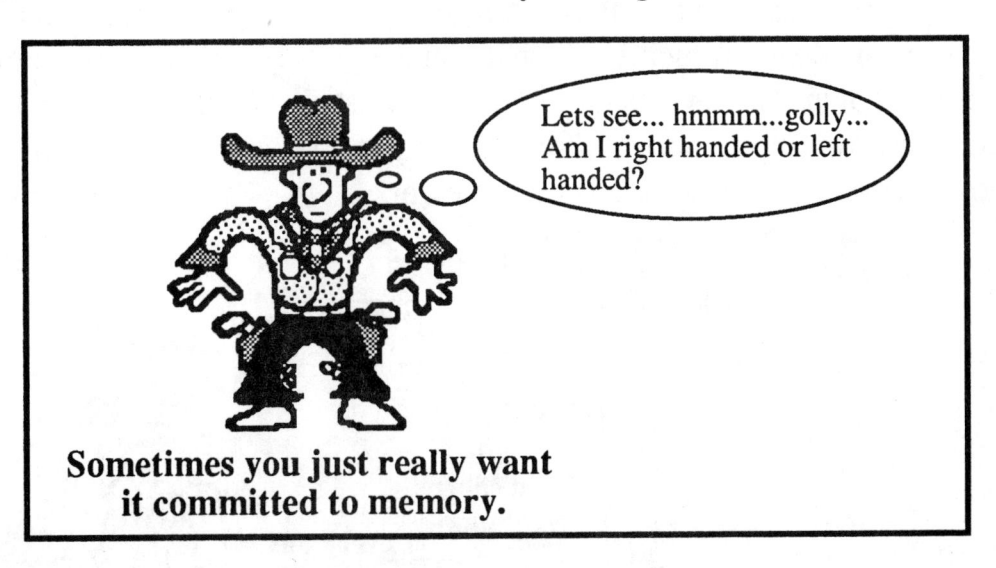

> Lets see... hmmm...golly... Am I right handed or left handed?
>
> **Sometimes you just really want it committed to memory.**

2) You must **do something active** like repeating it out loud, writing it, using flash cards, doing a recall pattern (you'll learn this technique next week), or simply repeat it in your mind over and over. Do this until you "overlearn" it.

Isn't that a lot of work?

Well, yes and no. It depends on what your goal is. If you want to learn a collection of important facts that will make your job *easier* as you go through school, this is essential. In the short run, it does take a little more time.

What If...

You worked to memorize a 30 line poem until you could say it perfectly *one time*. Would you still have it two months later? *No Way.*

Suppose that you had memorized the same poem perfectly once and then **overlearned** it by saying it 10 more times. Would you still have it six months later? *Probably yes,* and even if you didn't, it's likely that just a quick review would bring it back.

3) <u>Spread your memory practice</u> over several days. YOU WILL REMEMBER FAR MORE IF YOU MEMORIZE FOR 10 MINUTES A DAY FOR 5 DAYS THAN ONE DAY FOR 50 MINUTES. There is a good reason for this; memorizing information is *hard work* that is not particularly exciting. If you try to memorize for 50 minutes your mind will grow tired of the task and start to "float" in such a way that you are getting little benefit from the time you put in. However, short, frequent "bursts" of memorizing for 10-15 minutes are quite productive. Done this way, it is so easy that sometimes it's more pleasant than other kinds of homework.

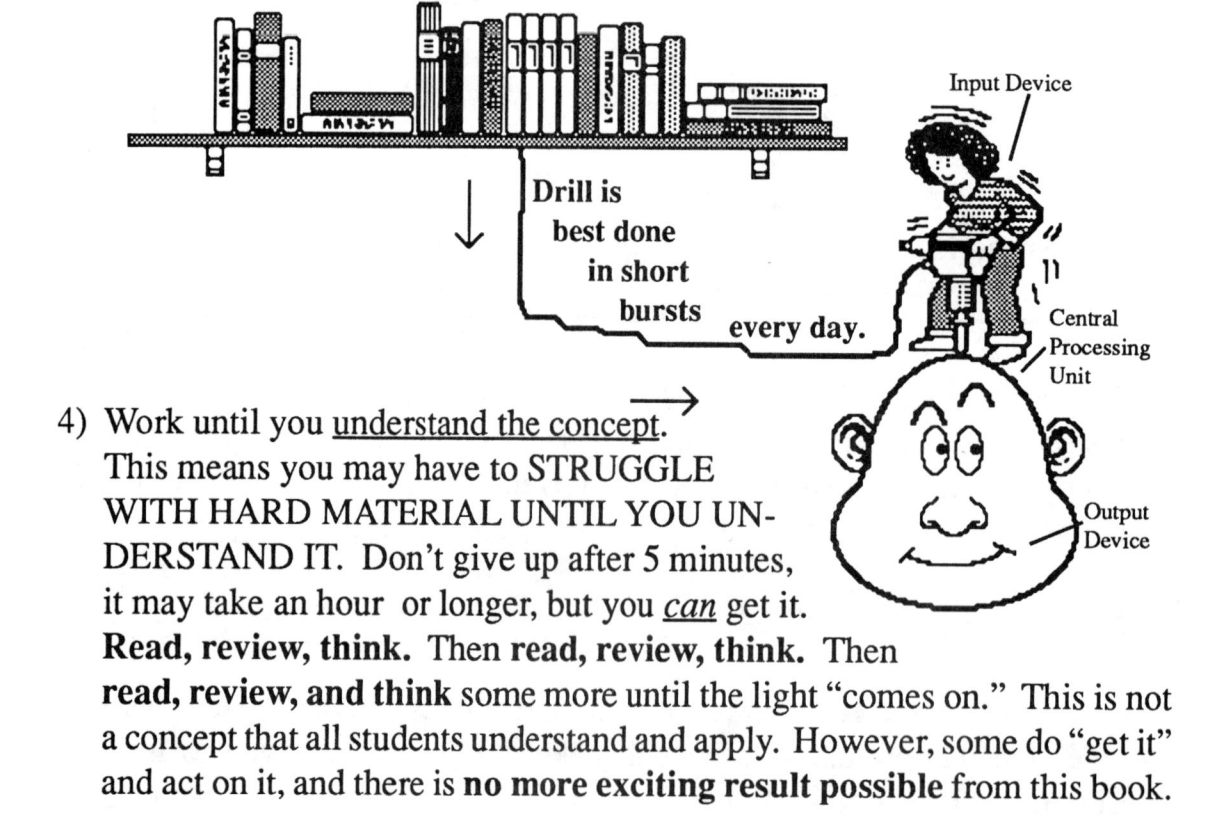

Drill is best done in short bursts every day.

4) Work until you <u>understand the concept</u>. This means you may have to STRUGGLE WITH HARD MATERIAL UNTIL YOU UNDERSTAND IT. Don't give up after 5 minutes, it may take an hour or longer, but you *can* get it. **Read, review, think.** Then **read, review, think.** Then **read, review, and think** some more until the light "comes on." This is not a concept that all students understand and apply. However, some do "get it" and act on it, and there is **no more exciting result possible** from this book.

To Tell the Truth...

When Ross was in graduate school, he took a course in Statistics at the Doctoral level. This is difficult stuff for nearly everybody. It demanded a very high level of concentration and hard work.

For example, when he first read a new chapter the sum total of his understanding was often the profound knowledge that it *looked like Greek*. $\Sigma \beta \Omega \partial \pi \emptyset$

The second reading his knowledge often vastly improved to understanding it was *about statistics*.

$$S^2 = \frac{\sum X^2 - \frac{(\sum X)^2}{N}}{N-1}$$

At the third reading he sensed that there was probably a thread of logic to it all. $E = MC^2$

At the fourth reading he began to understand it.   **Got it!**

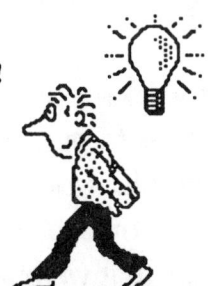

At the fifth and sixth readings, he worked on mastering it until he was confident about it. Then he reviewed it until it was automatic.

Final Exam 98%

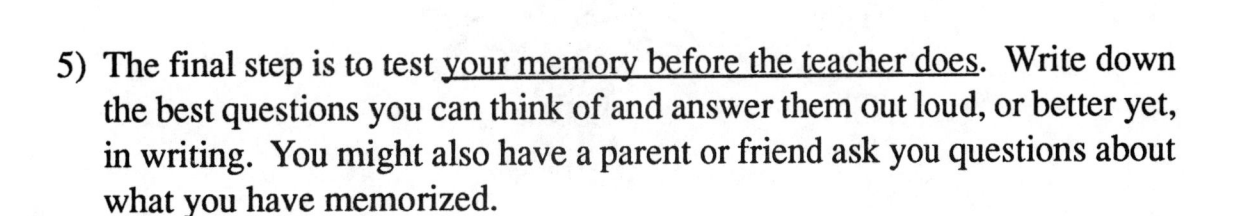

5) The final step is to test <u>your memory before the teacher does</u>. Write down the best questions you can think of and answer them out loud, or better yet, in writing. You might also have a parent or friend ask you questions about what you have memorized.

Mnemonic Devices (what they are and how to use them)

This odd and unusual looking word (mnemonic) is really not so bad. It simply means "Memory Trick." It comes from the Greek root word "mnemon" which means "mindful" (what a great way to describe a person who has made it a lifelong goal to remember things!) Human beings have been so "mindful" of the importance of good memory that there is even a Greek Goddess of memory named (what else?) Mnemosyne.

How to use Memory Tricks

Memory tricks are commonly used by just about everyone who goes very far in higher education. For example, doctors have a little jingle that helps them remember the little bones of the hand and wrist. Mnemonic devices work well to help you remember short facts of all kinds. It is a method used to "trigger" your memory.

Let's take a simple example. All of you probably memorized the 5 senses at one time. Can you say them all quickly? Go ahead and do it now.

If you are like many students in our workshops, you had a little trouble quickly remembering these senses. The trick is to put the information into a form that will "jog" your memory. For example, you might make a nonsense word "SHOTTS" which has the first letter of each word in it (S)ight, (H)earing, (T)ouch, (T)aste, and (S)mell. Notice that we put an extra "O" in the middle to make a nonsense word. It doesn't stand for anything, it's only there to help us make a more rememberable word.

Another way to use a mnemonic device is to put it in the form of a sentence by using the first letter of each word as the first letter of each word in the sentence. For example:

(S)ee
(H)im
(S)how
(T)he
(T)rout.

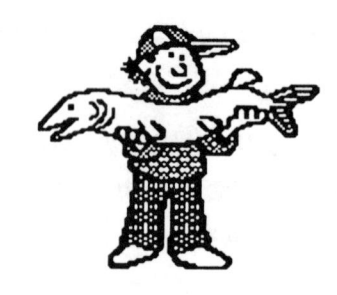

Special Assignment

This week we want you to practice **overlearning.** The most important feature will be that you **do something active.** What you are to do this week is to **tell yourself you will remember** what you read and **take handwritten notes** on at least one chapter from a book in social studies, English, or a science class. Your notes should be **very complete.** As a "ball park" figure, you should collect *at least* 6 pieces of information from each full page.

You are to do this reading in 3 steps:

1) **Carefully read** one section at a time (a section is often about a half to a whole page - you recognize them by their **bold headings**).

2) After you have read the section **close your book** and write down everything you can from memory (this is active learning).

3) When you can't think of anything more, open your book and **add anything you missed** to your notes.

When you are through, **overlearn** this information by *reading your notes over at least 4 times over a 2 day period.*

Few students understand the level of detail in studying that is necessary to really do your best. This week, you may learn something of great value.

To help you remember to do this, it will be one of the questions on your Checklist for next week.

Next comes the Checklist for this week.

The Checklist

(Parent and Student do together)

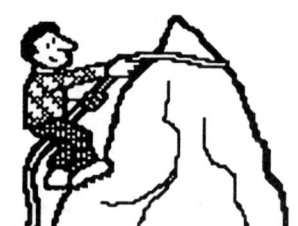

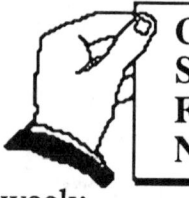

Continuing Special Focus: Notebook

Mark the following **yes** or **no** as was true of your week:

___ The student used the stopwatch and recorded accurate times at each study period.

___ The student is now using **a standard 3 ring notebook with divider tabs. All sections are arranged in logical order by subject and date.**

___ The student made his/her contracted study goal for the week or worked on Saturday morning until the contracted study time was made up. (Note: It is a parent responsibility to ask about this and to enforce it if necessary).

___ If the student has assignments that are not due immediately, he/she worked on them for at least 15 minutes each night or until they were done.

___ The student took the Study Plan to all teachers for comments once during the week. Low grades were compared with minutes spent on that subject during the past week and any needed time increases for next week were made and written into the Study Plan.

___ The student recorded every assignment, test, and quiz in the Assignment Sheet.

___ The student turned in every assignment this week.

___ The student took the Study Plan to his/her parent for their initials after every study period.

Next use the **Study Skills Summary**.

Study Skill Summary
Parent and Student do Together

1) **Negotiate the amount of study time** and enter it on a new **Study Plan** (a new Study Plan and Assignment Sheet are at the end of this chapter). Put the new Assignment Sheet and Study Plan at the *front of the student's regular school notebook* and be sure all school subjects are listed on the new Study Plan. Have your student **record his/her study time every day.** Parent's initial the Study Plan. **Don't skip the initials!** If your student didn't bring the Study Plan to you to initial last week, ask to see it each night.

2) If your student procrastinates, set a time to begin and allow 15 minutes and ONE SECOND leeway, then **assign an extra 20 minutes of homework**.

3) See that your student has a **quiet place to study** at a table or a desk. No TV, no radio, no stereo, no phone calls during study time.

4) The student **must use the stopwatch correctly.** NO EXCEPTIONS.

5) Check and **initial the assignment sheet daily** if your student is having trouble turning in assignments. If your child loses the assignment sheet or the study plan, begin a new one the same day. NO EXCEPTIONS!

6) Once a week, make sure your student gets a **teacher signature** for each academic class.

7) If you need extra support, **make an appointment** to talk with a teacher, counselor, or principal.

THERE IS NO SUCH THING AS NOT HAVING HOMEWORK! The only students who say this are underachieving. Remember, the student can (a) study ahead or behind and/or rework assignments, (b) ask teachers for help and/or extra credit to fill up homework time, and (c) check out three books related to his/her subjects from the library to read during study time.

Parents may also know that the student needs to work on certain weaknesses and may assign the student a particular task. For example, parents may require their student to work on math facts, vocabulary, spelling lists, or independent reading.

Go over Your Checklist

Now, return to your Checklist on page 67 and make a plan with your student to correct any of the questions that were answered "no." **◁ Do it now**

You should have already negotiated the amount of study time the student will study and the student should have **written it into the Study Plan.** If for any reason this hasn't been done, do it now.

You are now set for the coming week.

If either of you are even a little concerned that you may have a misunderstanding about your exact agreement, you may write your plan below.

_____

_____

_____

_____

_____

STOP

This is the end of Week Four. On the next two pages are a new **Study Plan** and **Assignment Sheet.** You may use these this week but *do not* go to the next chapter, Week Five, until you have studied for one week. However, do be sure to **plan** the day of the week you will read Week Five and mark it on your home calendar. See you next week!

Study Plan
Academic Skills Workshop

Name: _____

Date: _____

Daily Goals

Subjects:						Week Total	Teacher Comments: Grade/Attitude/All Work Turned In?
Total Stopwatch Time For All Subjects:							
When Did You Start?						WEEKLY AVERAGE = _____ Minutes/Day	
When Did You Finish?						(Add total number of minutes for the week and divide by 5 days.)	
Place You Studied:							
Parent's Initials:							

COPYRIGHT © **January 1, 1988 by Counseling and Workshop Professionals**
Unauthorized Reproductions Are Illegal and may be Punishable by Large Fines.
Students who have individually purchased this book may make copies for their own personal use. Copies may not be made for friends. School Districts are **Expressly Forbidden** to replicate these materials. A special discount is available to schools. Call (503) 588-1010 for ordering information.

Assignment Sheet

Write down the exact assignment before leaving class

Class	Assignment	Date Given	Date Due	Date Turned In	Parent Initials

Week 5

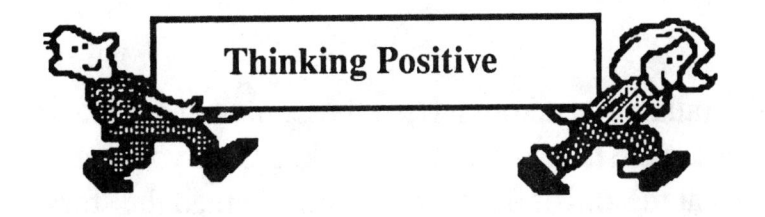

Thinking Positive

Thinking Positive

Welcome to week 5!

This week we want to talk about attitude. Some things are under our control, while others aren't. The famed Jewish psychiatrist, Victor Frankl, who spent years as a victim and witness to mankind's inhumanity to man in Nazi concentration camps during World War II, emerged to share a profound understanding with the rest of the world: in any given circumstance we may not be able to control what is happening to us, but we do have control over our attitude toward it.

In this country we have incredible freedom to choose our own direction as we mature. And like our faces, the older we grow, the more responsible we become for ourselves and the way things turned out. In the beginning, each of us received the gift of life and a set of potentials that came with it. Each of us has an obligation to develop the potential and become the best person we can be.

But . . .

some of us take rather odd detours to get there. In my case (Ross), I had to learn an important lesson the hard way. This week, before you analyze *your* detours on the Checklist at the end of the chapter, you can read the story of an academic disaster that allowed me to finally start growing up.

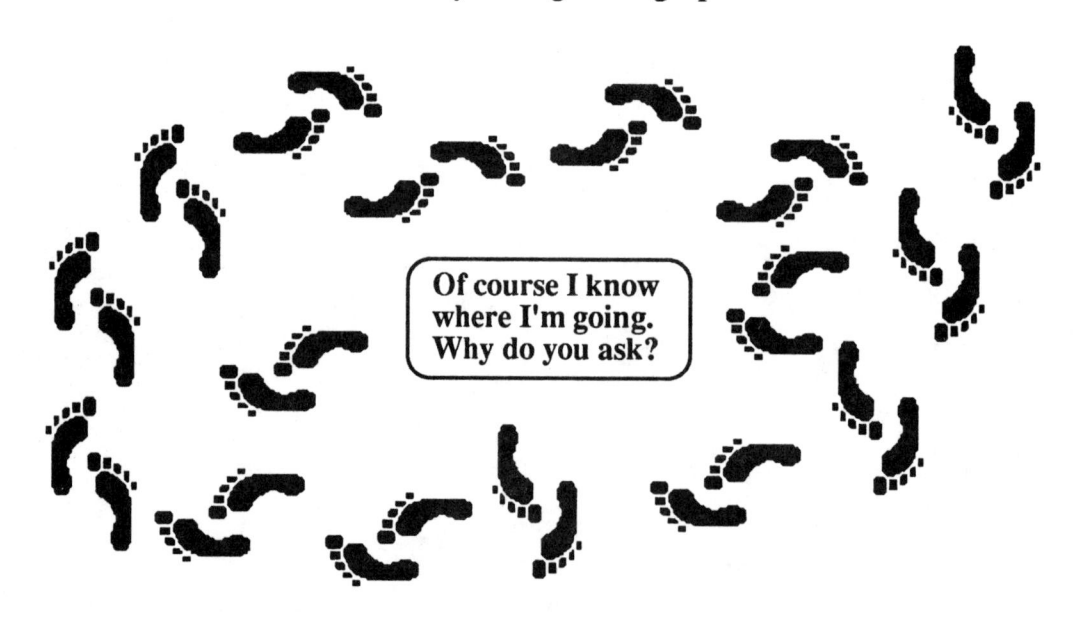

Of course I know where I'm going. Why do you ask?

The Rise and Fall of Western Civilization

I arrived at a small liberal arts college as freshman in the Fall of '68. It was a rebellious time for students in the country as a whole and while I was never radical, I did entertain some rather presumptuous attitudes and opinions. Not the least of which was that I felt it was **unfair** to have to take **required courses.** After all, wasn't I the best judge of what was good for me?

Well, in particular, I didn't think I should have to take a course in the *History of Western Civilization* required of all freshman (I would probably "kill" to do it now). My attitude was lousy, but I did have the presence of mind to sign up in advance for a class from a professor who had a good reputation. You couldn't switch classes after a cut-off date. However, **after the cut-off date,** this professor was pulled from the course (I think he died or something), and the college substituted a man *at the last minute* who was from the Office of Admissions who had never taught the course before! Well, THAT DID IT. I couldn't change the class, and I felt ripped-off about having to take it in the first place.

I showed up for the class expecting the worst. And of course I found it. The professor was overweight, smiled wrong, talked too much, made odd hand gestures, passed out post cards of Europe, and I didn't like the textbook. Strangely, I don't remember him being angry, unfair, or demeaning, but then in those days I apparently had different standards for appraising people.

Over the next few weeks I made it a point to show up late for class. Being a psychology major, I felt very clever to point out all of his various "defects" to the people with the "good fortune" to sit next to me. From the response I got, I soon discovered that I was apparently in *sole possession* of this vital information. Of course this made me feel even more important and clever. After the 4th week I decided that as a matter of principle I wouldn't go to the class except when *I* wanted to, and take the mid-term and the final. It was *my life* right?

> What do you mean BAD ATTITUDE?!

Right. Well, I got what I deserved, a "D-" if memory serves me well. I also found a few "nasty" comments on my grade slip to the effect that **he really didn't think my problem was intelligence.** He just thought I had a **lousy attitude** and it would have helped if I had come to class more often.

Boy, was I furious. What right did *he* have to judge *me?* But after a week I calmed down and I had two extremely important insights that I carried with me for my next 10 years of education.

Insight 1: **Guess who <u>always</u> loses when a student gets into a power struggle with a teacher?** The student. In fact, it really hurt my ego, but about 6 months later I realized that he *probably didn't even know he was in a power struggle with me.*

Insight 2: It was true what he said about my intelligence, it wasn't so low that my potential was achieved with a "D-." That left only my **attitude** to ponder. *I resolved never to let that happen again.*

Today I am grateful to that professor because I learned a great deal in his class; it just wasn't about Western Civilization.

The Next Challenge: Italian Renaissance Painting

I remembered this little lesson when I walked into another course I "had to take" - *Italian Renaissance Painting* - about which I knew nothing. When I went to the first class I was dismayed that the professor was probably about 70 years old, mumbled *and* rambled when he talked, and didn't respond to questions well. When he showed us paintings, he spoke with great reverence about perspective, texture, color, shading, light and so on. Which worried me greatly because all I could see was a lot of fairly nice religious paintings but I wouldn't put them on *my* wall. One Madonna and Child looked pretty much like the next Madonna and Child to me no matter who painted it. To make matters worse, the class was full of beginning Art Majors who seemed to understand what he was talking about. Then I learned that each student had to study the work of one artist in detail and give a one hour presentation to the whole class. At this point I really did know the truth: *my life was over!*

This was a perfect **set-up** to write off the course as irrelevant as I had *Western Civilization*.

But I was determined not to this time. In fact, I decided I *would find something about the course that I could like and understand.* So I went to the library that first week and **started searching early** (before anyone else) for the artist I would present. I even tried talking out loud to myself about the perspective, texture, color, shading and use of light of several artists. However, I knew I didn't know what I was talking about and it sounded so funny coming out of my mouth it made me laugh.

But then a really great thing happened; I found Leonardo da Vinci. And since I had started early, I wasn't in a hurry just to "get something done." So I allowed myself to read about his science and life first. Here was something I could understand and marvel over. A man of unsurpassed genius born at a time in history when this great mind and talent could dominate science and art at the same time. In the 15th Century he had conceived airplanes that were accurately designed to fly if engines were known, the helicopter, the parachute, and scuba diving gear. He was variously described as:

* **A Painter**
* **A Sculptor**
* **An Architect**
* **A Military and Hydraulic Engineer**
* **An Inventor**
* **An Anatomist**
* **A Naturalist**
* **A Musician**

The more I read, the more deeply engrossed I became. As I read page after page of inventions and science I lost track of time. Suddenly, I turned a page and there was the Mona Lisa. And I *appreciated an Italian Renaissance painting for the first time.*

The next day, I went to the Art professor and told him that I had spent several hours in the library and had settled on Leonardo da Vinci for my presentation. I was the first to choose a painter so he was pleased. I then told him the truth about my lack of understanding of the finer points of painting and asked if I could just present his science. At this he was less pleased, but he could see that

I really *was* trying and that I probably didn't have the potential to be one of his "star" Art Majors anyway. He reluctantly agreed but told me it would not be possible to get an "A" for a presentation so removed from the true subject matter of the course. That was OK with me. I was worried about PASSING pure and simple.

The rest is history. I worked with real enjoyment on that presentation and actually had fun giving it to the class. I don't believe I have ever been more pleased with a "B+" on an assignment in all of my years in school. The best part was the knowing deep down that I had mastered my own attitude and found a way to make a difficult, "boring" subject so exciting that even now I experience pleasure thinking about it.

> The moral of these two stories, is that **it is just about impossible to learn when you have a bad attitude.** It is always possible to find *something* about the instructor or the course that you can like and focus on that to pull you through.

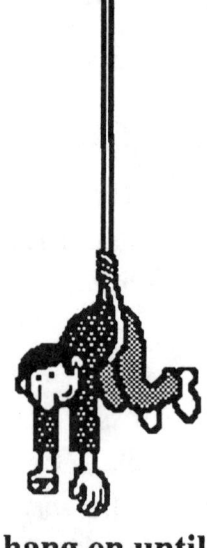

Just hang on until you find something to like.

Common Problems and Solutions

Problem 1: The student is telling you it is not important to use the stopwatch anymore.

The Solution : The reason students want to stop using the stopwatch is because they are not accustomed to such a high level of accountability. It focuses the issue *every night*. It is a **major mistake to stop.**

Problem 2: The student assures you it is no longer necessary to take their **Study Plan** to teachers once a week.

The Solution: Until your student solidly demonstrates that he/she is really out of danger in *all* classes, it is extremely important to keep doing this. At a minimum, we would keep this expectation if there are any "D" or "F" grades *or* the student is still not turning in **all** assignments on time.

Problem 3: Your student has gotten sloppy about filling out the Assignment Sheet.

The Solution: This too is an accountability issue - and a **very important one** at that. We expect students to continue to do this as long as they are in school. Before parents sign off on the **Study Plan** each night they must also check the assignment sheet, make eye contact, and ask if everything is recorded.

Assignment Sheet

Write down the exact assignment before leaving class

Class	Assignment	Date Given	Date Due	Date Turned In	Parent Initial

Make eye contact and ask!

Problem 4: You expect your child's grades to improve faster than they are.

The Solution: What your child has control over is effort, the teacher has control over grades. As long as your child is working hard *be supportive whatever the outcome.* (We once took a phone call from a mother who complained that her daughter had a 2.98 G.P.A. and "she needed a 3.0 to get into college." She wanted to know if it was "essential" that her daughter take our workshop. On further questioning we learned that the daughter studied hard nearly every night for two hours and always turned things in on time. Now, who really has the problem here?)

Next you will learn a very important skill: How to read a textbook for recall.

How to Read a Textbook for Recall

To introduce this section properly we must first tell you a little bit about how a human brain works. This will be gross oversimplification and we apologize in advance to any neurologists in the crowd, but we have an practical point to make. First, look at the diagram below. The perspective is from the top, looking down on a human head, with the top cut away. You say it doesn't look exactly like that? Looks more like a turtle or a bug? Use your imagination. Thanks.

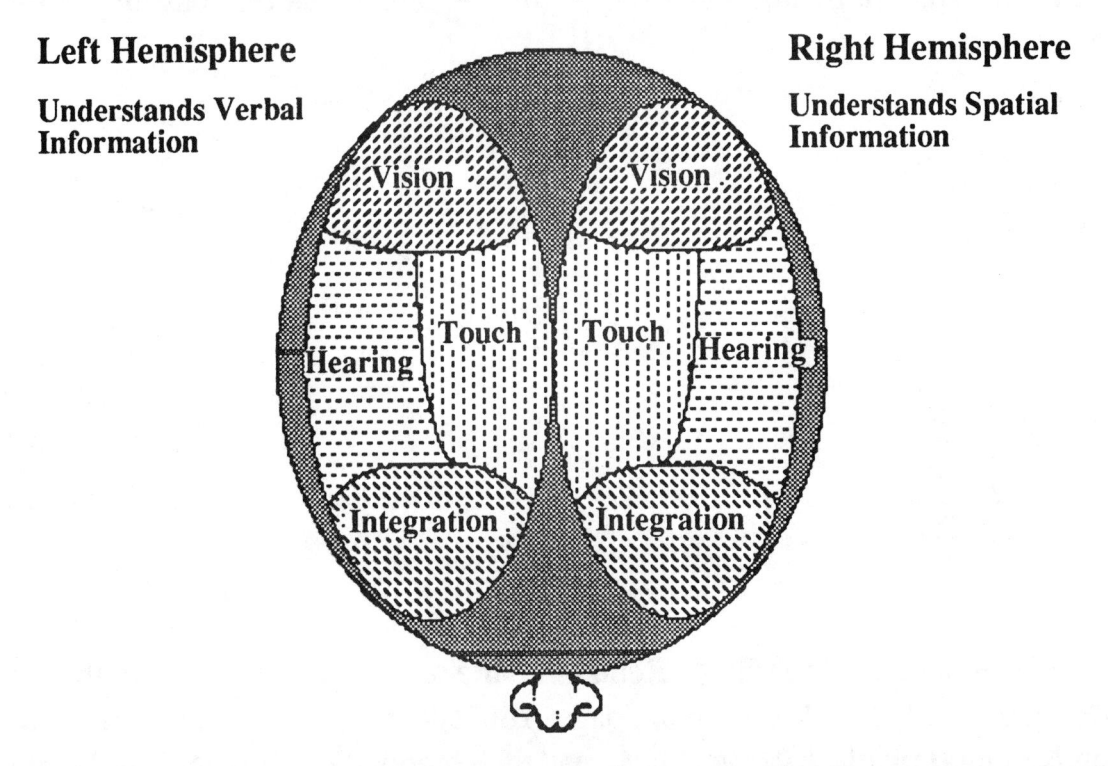

Left Hemisphere

Understands Verbal Information

Right Hemisphere

Understands Spatial Information

Notice that different senses are processed in different parts of the brain. For example, vision is in the back (occipital lobes), touch is on the top (parietal lobes), hearing is on the sides (temporal lobes), and integration occurs in the front (frontal lobes).

When you listen, your temporal lobes are activated. When you read, your occipital lobes are activated. When you write, your parietal lobes are activated. When you integrate and plan things, your frontal lobes are activated. When you study, the best chance you have of comprehending and remembering is when **you activate all these brain regions at the same time.** *Perhaps you can see right away that when you "passively read" that information doesn't have much chance at getting stored in your temporal lobes (hearing) or parietal lobes (writing).*

Yet, this is how most junior and senior high students study.

Making **Recall Patterns** and saying the information you write down is a powerful way to integrate and remember information because it taps all 4 of these brain areas. It is done in 3 steps:

Step 1: *Do a quick preview* of the entire chapter (2-3 minutes) and write down the **Title** of the chapter in the middle of a page and then put in the **Major Sections.** All you are doing at this point is making a "blueprint" of the material to be learned. Following is an example of how a recall pattern on study skills might start.

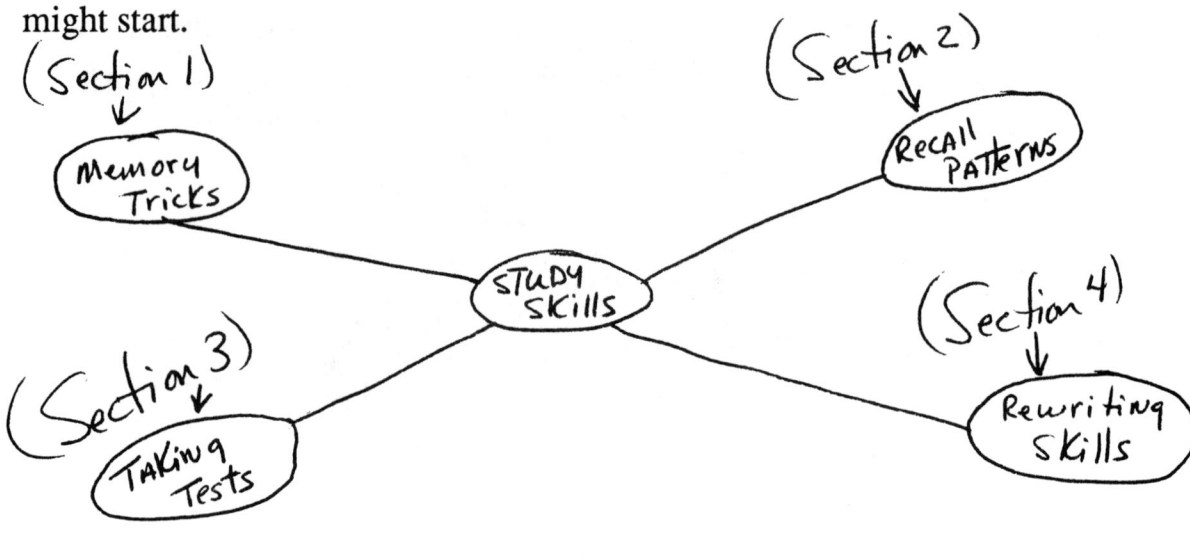

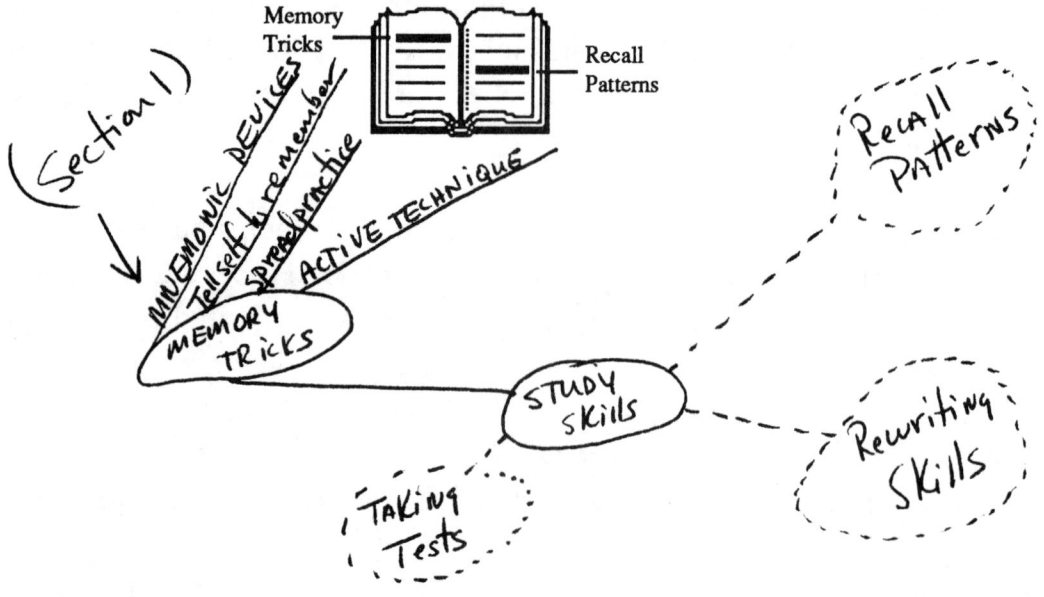

Step 2: Do a careful reading. Read only one section at a time. In textbooks there are usually 1 or 2 sections to a page. You recognize them because the heading is in **bold print.** After you have read the section, **close the book** and write

down all you can from memory on your recall pattern (this is *active* learning). See below.

Step 3: Review with your book open and write down anything you missed.
Do this each time you finish a section and continue this for each section until the chapter is finished. See below.

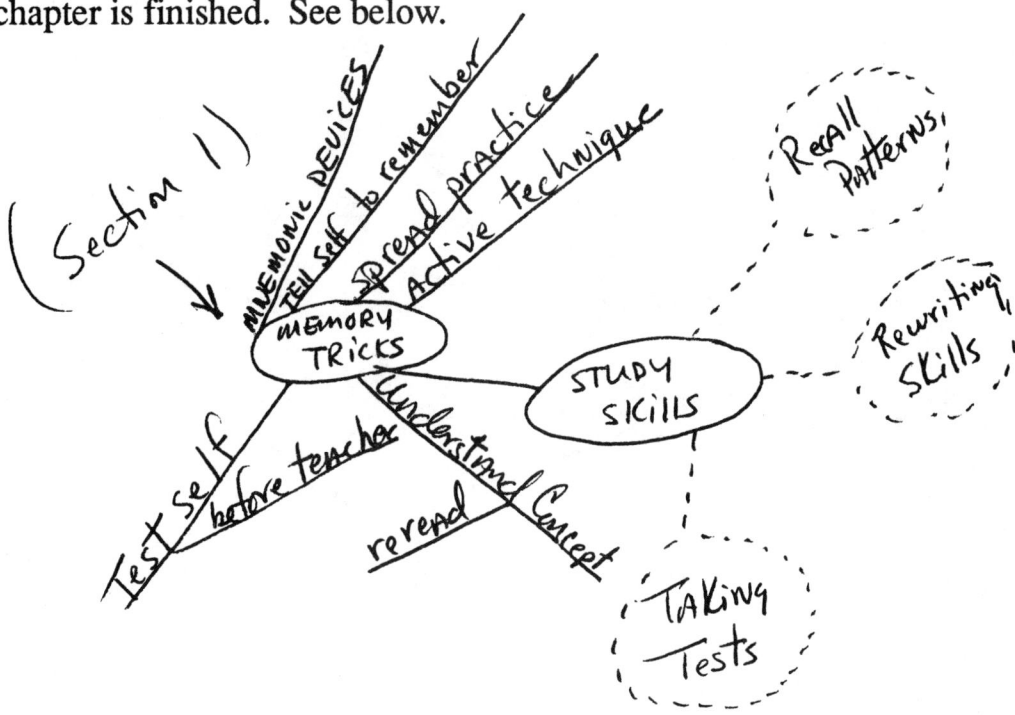

[Hand-drawn recall pattern diagram with central node "MEMORY TRICKS" (labeled "Section 1") connected to branches: MNEMONIC DEVICES, Tell self to remember, Spread practice, Active technique, Understand concept, reread, Test self before teacher. Connected to "STUDY SKILLS" node with dashed branches to "Recall Patterns", "Rewriting Skills", and "Taking Tests".]

When you are done with section one, go on to section two, and so on. Thus, to summarize, the steps go:

Preview the chapter and make an outline (step one). Then...

Read Carefully   **Close Book, Write What You Remember**   **Open Book and Add to Recall Pattern**

On the next page is the finished example of an excellent recall pattern done by a student who really understood how to make this work for him. His social studies test score jumped about 2 whole letter grades when he did this pattern. Three years later, we ran into his mother at a lecture about study skills we gave to parents at a local middle school. She was pleased to report that the improvement he made during the workshop stayed with him.

A "Star" Recall Pattern

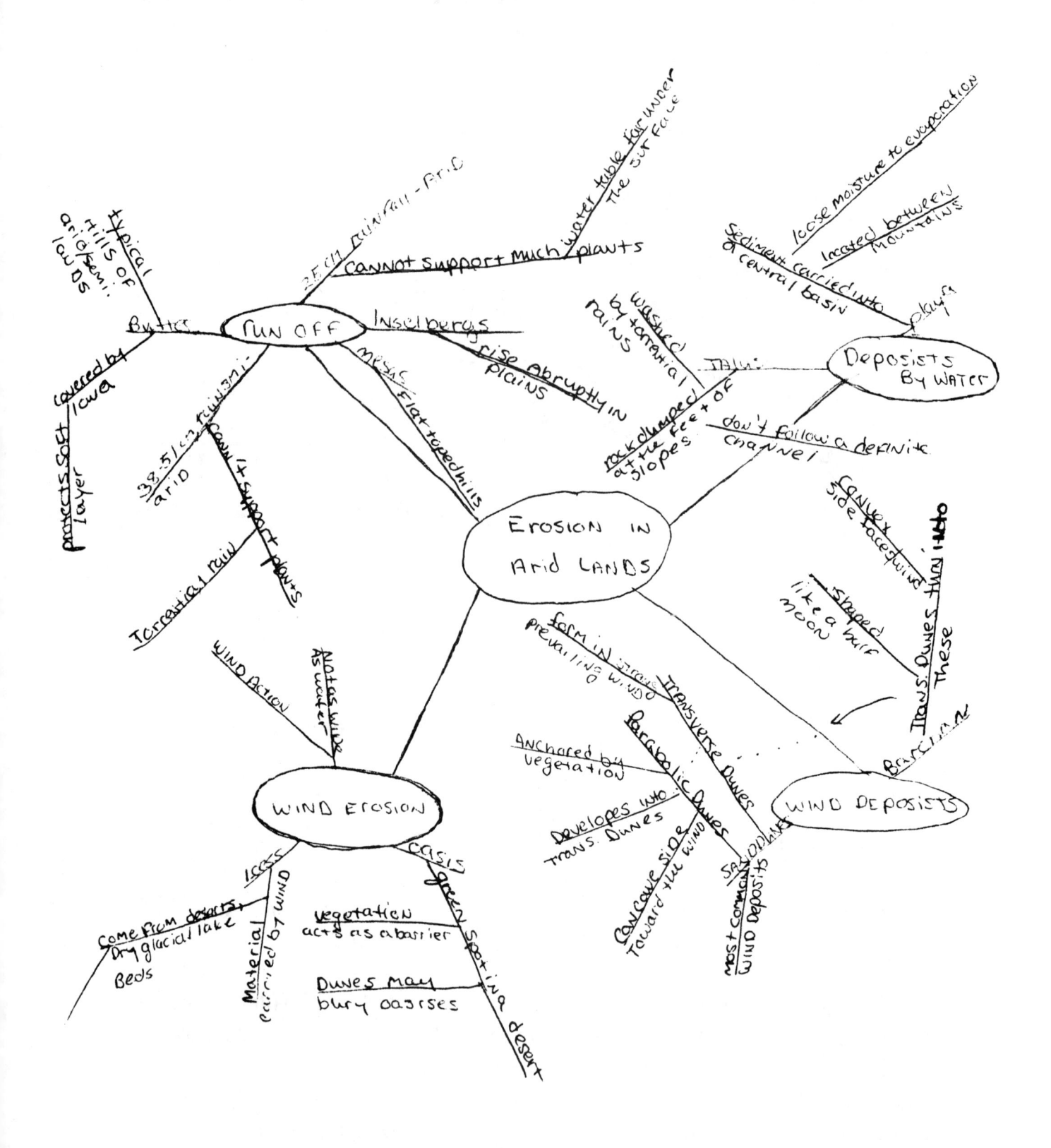

83

Setting Up a Recall Pattern for a Test.

Some students who have been through our Workshops have been able to improve test scores by a whole grade **just by preparing with recall patterns.** You will be most efficient if you *estimate* how many questions will be on the test. This may be difficult, but *any intelligent guess is better than none.* Suppose you guess there will be 20 questions (many teachers are quite predictable). What you must do is double the amount of information you put on your recall pattern to 40 pieces (20 x 2 = 40). This is because what you think is important, and what the teacher thinks is important may be different. So you need to plan ahead to remember *twice as much information* as you think will be on the test.

Now, if you need to record 40 facts, the way to use recall patterns most effectively is to write down an *equal number of facts in each of the main sections* of your recall pattern. This will help you find what is important in every section of the chapter - which is difficult for many students. For example, if there are 4 sections then you would record 10 pieces of informations in each one (4 x 10 = 40), like this:

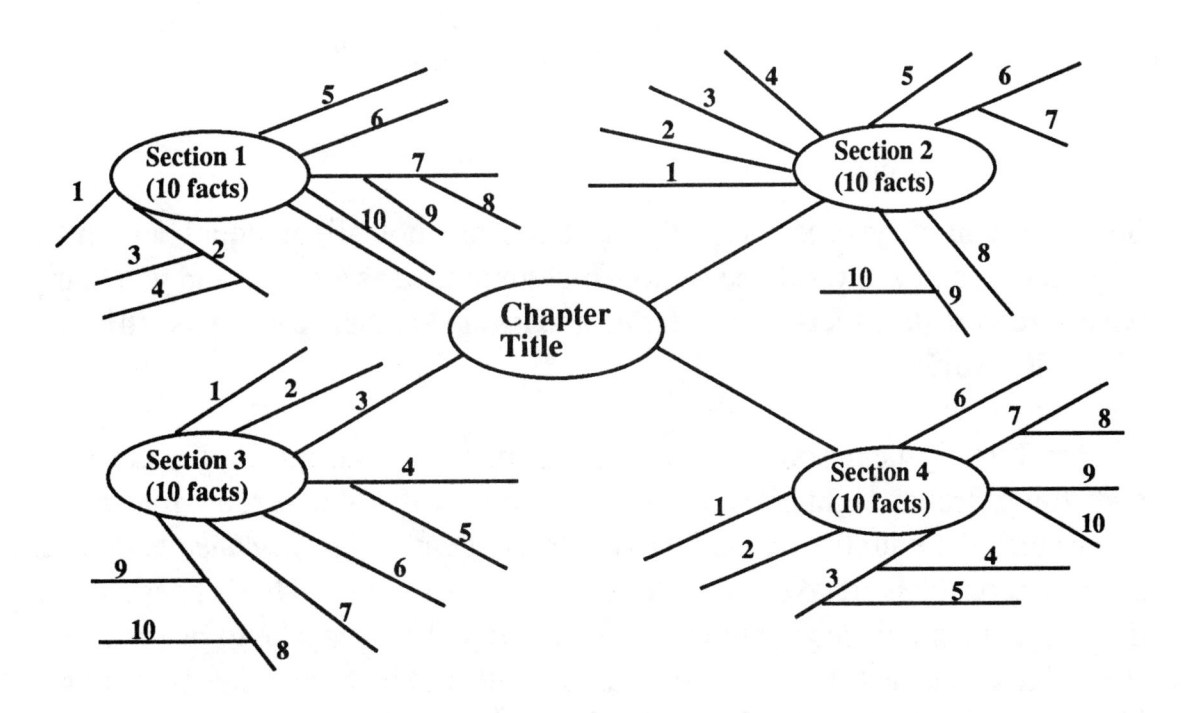

To give you another example, if there were 5 main sections and you needed 40 pieces of information you would write 8 facts in each section (5 x 8 = 40).

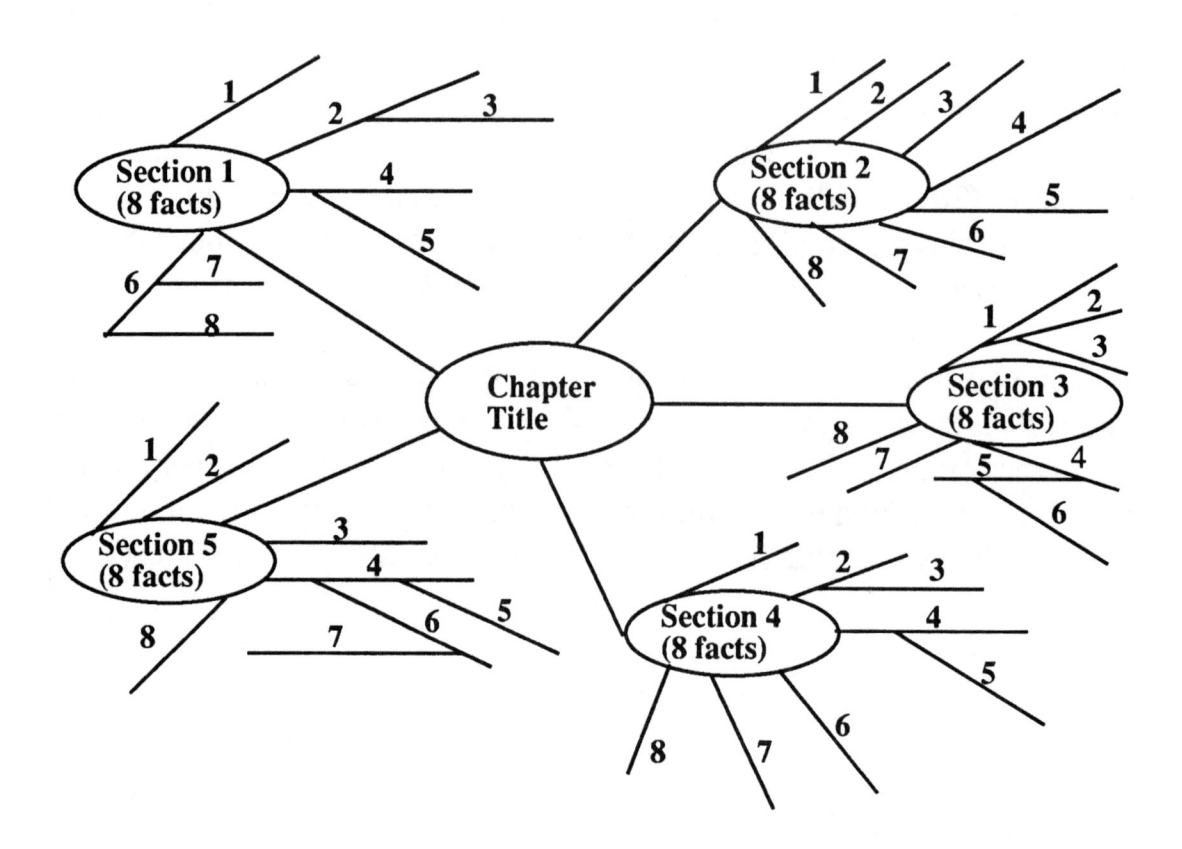

Some of you may object that the sections are not all of equal length or importance, and you would be right. This is intended as a guide, and you many wish to record more facts in one section and less in another. **But do use this tool - it really works!**

We can already hear some of you saying this will take too long. Let's set something straight right here. The actual writing will not take more than about 10 minutes. The study of material to the *level of detail that you need to do well on tests* probably will take you an "extra" 30 to 40 minutes. This is because you do not have a good idea about just how long it really does take to be prepared. If you have been getting low scores on tests, it's not that this takes "too long," it's that *you haven't studied to the right level of detail before.*

A Final Note on Recall Patterns

Many students might prefer to take more traditional outline notes on the material they read (as you did in the previous chapter). However, we want you to try this method **at least once this week.** This is because we think that it allows the right brain hemisphere (which understands spatial information) to *see a pattern* which seems to help some students remember. As a result, some students seem to be able to close their eyes on test day and mentally "trace" the recall pattern until they find the information they want. At a minimum, recall patterns *group related information together* which helps with memory.

Special Assignment

All students are to discuss with their parent *right now* which class they will use to do a recall pattern. **◄ Do it Now** You may want to select a class in which you have a test so you can really try it out. Also, some students find the task more enjoyable if they use different colors to make it. That's fine. To help you remember to get this done, **it will be on your Checklist** for next week.

Remember, (1) **Preview** and set up main sections, (2) **Careful Read** then close the book and write down what you remember, and (3) **Review** by opening the book and writing down what you missed.

Read Carefully One Section at a Time

Close Book, Write What You Remember

Open Book, Review, and Add to Recall Pattern

Next read over the **Checklist.**

The Checklist

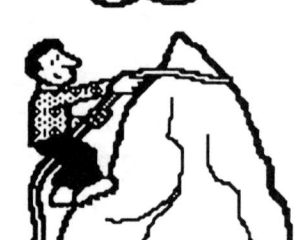

(Parent and Student do together)

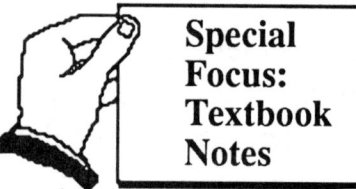

Special Focus: Textbook Notes

Mark the following **yes** or **no** as was true of your week:

___ **The student practiced overlearning by taking complete notes on at least on chapter from a textbook.**

___ The student used the stopwatch and recorded accurate times at each study period.

___ The student is now using a standard 3 ring notebook with divider tabs. All sections are arranged in logical order by subject and date.

___ The student made his/her contracted study goal for the week or worked on Saturday morning until the contracted study time was made up. (Note: It is a parent responsibility to ask about this and to enforce it if necessary).

___ If the student has assignments that are not due immediately, he/she worked on them 15 minutes each night or until they were done.

___ The student took the Study Plan to all teachers for comments once during the week. Low grades were compared with minutes spent on that subject during the past week and any needed time increases for next week were made and written into the Study Plan.

___ The student recorded every assignment, test, and quiz in the Assignment Sheet.

___ The student turned in every assignment this week.

___ The student took the Study Plan to his/her parent for their initials after every study period.

Next, turn to the **Study Skills Summary**.

Study Skill Summary
Parent and Student do Together

1) **Negotiate the amount of study time** and enter it on a new **Study Plan** (a new Study Plan and Assignment Sheet are at the end of this chapter). Put the new Assignment Sheet and Study Plan at the *front of the student's regular school notebook* and be sure all school subjects are listed on the new Study Plan. Have your student **record his/her study time every day.** Parent's initial the Study Plan. **Don't skip the initials!** If your student didn't bring the Study Plan to you to initial last week, ask to see it each night.

2) If your student procrastinates, set a time to begin and allow 15 minutes and ONE SECOND leeway, then **assign an extra 20 minutes of homework.**

3) See that your student has a **quiet place to study** at a table or a desk. No TV, no radio, no stereo, no phone calls during study time.

4) The student **must use the stopwatch correctly.** NO EXCEPTIONS.

5) Check and **initial the assignment sheet daily** if your student is having trouble turning in assignments. If your child loses the assignment sheet or the study plan, begin a new one the same day. NO EXCEPTIONS!

6) Once a week, make sure your student gets a **teacher signature** for each academic class.

7) If you need extra support, **make an appointment** to talk with a teacher, counselor, or principal.

THERE IS NO SUCH THING AS NOT HAVING HOMEWORK! The only students who say this are underachieving. Remember, the student can (a) study ahead or behind and/or rework assignments, (b) ask teachers for help and/or extra credit to fill up homework time, and (c) check out three books related to his/her subjects from the library to read during study time.

Parents may also know that the student needs to work on certain weaknesses and may assign the student a particular task. For example, parents may require their student to work on math facts, vocabulary, spelling lists, or independent reading.

Go over Your Checklist

Now, return to your Checklist on page 87 and make a plan with your student to correct any of the questions that were answered "no." **◀ Do it Now**

You should have already negotiated the amount of study time the student will study and the student should have **written it into the new Study Plan.** If for any reason this hasn't been done, do it now.

You are now set for the coming week.

If either of you are even a little concerned that you may have a misunderstanding about your exact agreement, you may write your plan below.

_____

_____

_____

_____

_____

STOP

This is the end of Week Five. On the next two pages are a new **Study Plan** and **Assignment Sheet.** You may use these this week but *do not* go to the next chapter, Week Six, until you have studied for one week.
However, do be sure to **plan** the day of the week you will read Week Six and mark it on your home calendar.
See you next week!

Study Plan
Academic Skills Workshop

Name: _____

Date: _____

Daily Goals

Subjects:						Week Total	Teacher Comments: Grade/Attitude/All Work Turned In?
Total Stopwatch Time For All Subjects:						WEEKLY AVERAGE = _____ Minutes/Day (Add total number of minutes for the week and divide by 5 days.)	
When Did You Start?							
When Did You Finish?							
Place You Studied:							
Parent's Initials:							

COPYRIGHT © January 1, 1988 by Counseling and Workshop Professionals

Unauthorized Reproductions Are Illegal and may be Punishable by Large Fines.

Students who have individually purchased this book may make copies for their own personal use. Copies may not be made for friends. School Districts are **Expressly Forbidden** to replicate these materials. A special discount is available to schools. Call (503) 588-1010 for ordering information.

Assignment Sheet

Write down the exact assignment before leaving class

Class	Assignment	Date Given	Date Due	Date Turned In	Parent Initials

Week 6

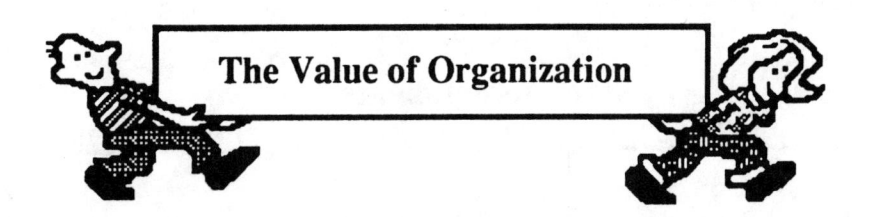

The Value of Organization

The Value of Organization

Over and over again we have stressed the importance of turning work in. Being able to turn work in is the end product of lots of organization. If you think about it for a moment, there are quite a few steps involved:

1) You go to class.
2) Your teacher gives you an assignment.
3) You write it down.
4) You remember to take it home and include the right books/materials.
5) You spend time and effort to complete the assignment.
6) You remember to take it back to school with you.
7) The teacher asks for it.
8) You have it with you and turn it in.

Is it all worth it? **You bet it is!** The following information was put together by a high school mathematics department. It shows a very interesting relationship between grades in the first semester and the percentage of assignments that were turned in and the number of days absent. Take a look:

Grade	% of Assignments Turned In	Days Absent
A	96%	4
B	89%	5
C	83%	7
D	69%	8
F	53%	16

As you can see, there is an incredibly strong relationship. The students who got "A's" turned in nearly all of their work on time while students who got "F's" only turned in a little over 1/2 of the assignments.

We suspect that there is little, if any, difference in intelligence that separates a "C" student from an "F" student. The main difference is probably that a "C" student is turning in about 4 out of 5 assignments and goes to school fairly regularly while the "F" student only gets about 1 out of 2 turned in and is absent from school twice as often as the "C" student.

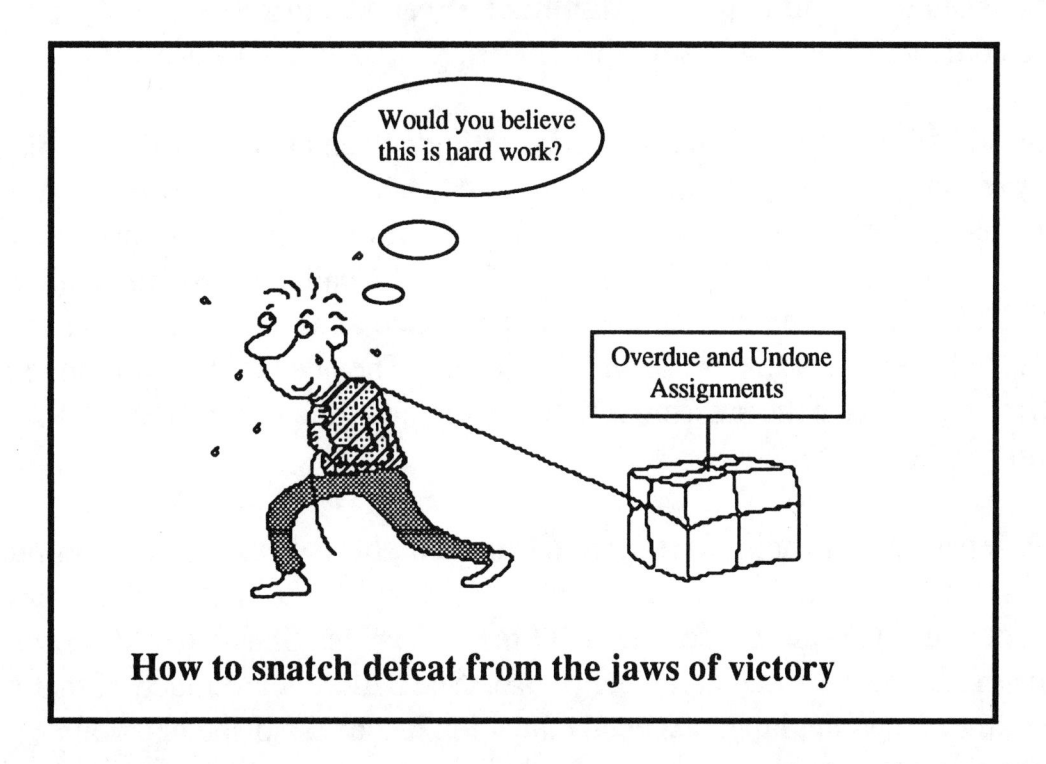

How to snatch defeat from the jaws of victory

Next, read about a student who really didn't need to fail, but nearly stayed **Dedicated to Failure.**

Dedicated to Failure?

Jerry was running a group for failing students at his high school. It was held during school hours and parents were not involved. Jenny, a sophomore, wasn't getting any better. In fact, she was getting more resistant and angry:

If Jerry said to study 5 days, she did 2 or 3.
If he said to get all the teachers signatures, she got 1 out of 5.
If he asked her to fill out the **Assignment Sheet,** she lost it.
If he confronted her, she'd say it was "boring" and "who needs this?"

It got so bad that her passive/aggressive attitude began to affect the other kids. Jerry reluctantly decided that he would have to take her out of the group. When he called her parents to tell them about his decision, he found out that she was dyslexic for the first time. When he heard that, he called Jenny out again and individually discussed her reading problem. She admitted that she had been trying to hide her reading problem in the group. They decided to work together individually to take the pressure off. Jenny seemed relieved and began to smile again for the first time in weeks.

With Jerry's private help, she began to study 5 nights a week for 30-45 minutes almost immediately. The result was that at the end of the first grading period, she got some C's and B's for the first time in 3 years. She also told Jerry that some of her teachers had given her praise. She hadn't heard much of that in a long time. In particular, her special education teacher said she had done a real turnaround and was showing some pride in her work for the first time.

A few weeks later, the special education teacher was doing a class on goal setting. Another student said his goal was to improve his grades. Jenny told him, "if you want to improve your grades, go see Mr. Gastineau and do the Academic Skills Program."

She had gone from belligerent to supportive in 5 weeks.

I learned something that changed my attitude.

Reflection:

We think that all schools should have a structured program to help kids improve their school performance. If nothing else, the relationship between turning work in and getting better grades is so clear that it should be the cornerstone of any attempt to help students. While teachers clearly have a *critical role* to play in providing a stimulating classroom and requiring accountability, they cannot do it all. Classrooms that average 25-30 children are unrealistically high to provide sufficient individualized attention. **Many potentially successful students "fall between the cracks."** This is especially true at the junior and senior high levels when teachers might easily have 6 classes per day and the responsibility to track as many as 120 to 150 students per day! Simply remembering names and grading/recording assignments is a big job in itself.

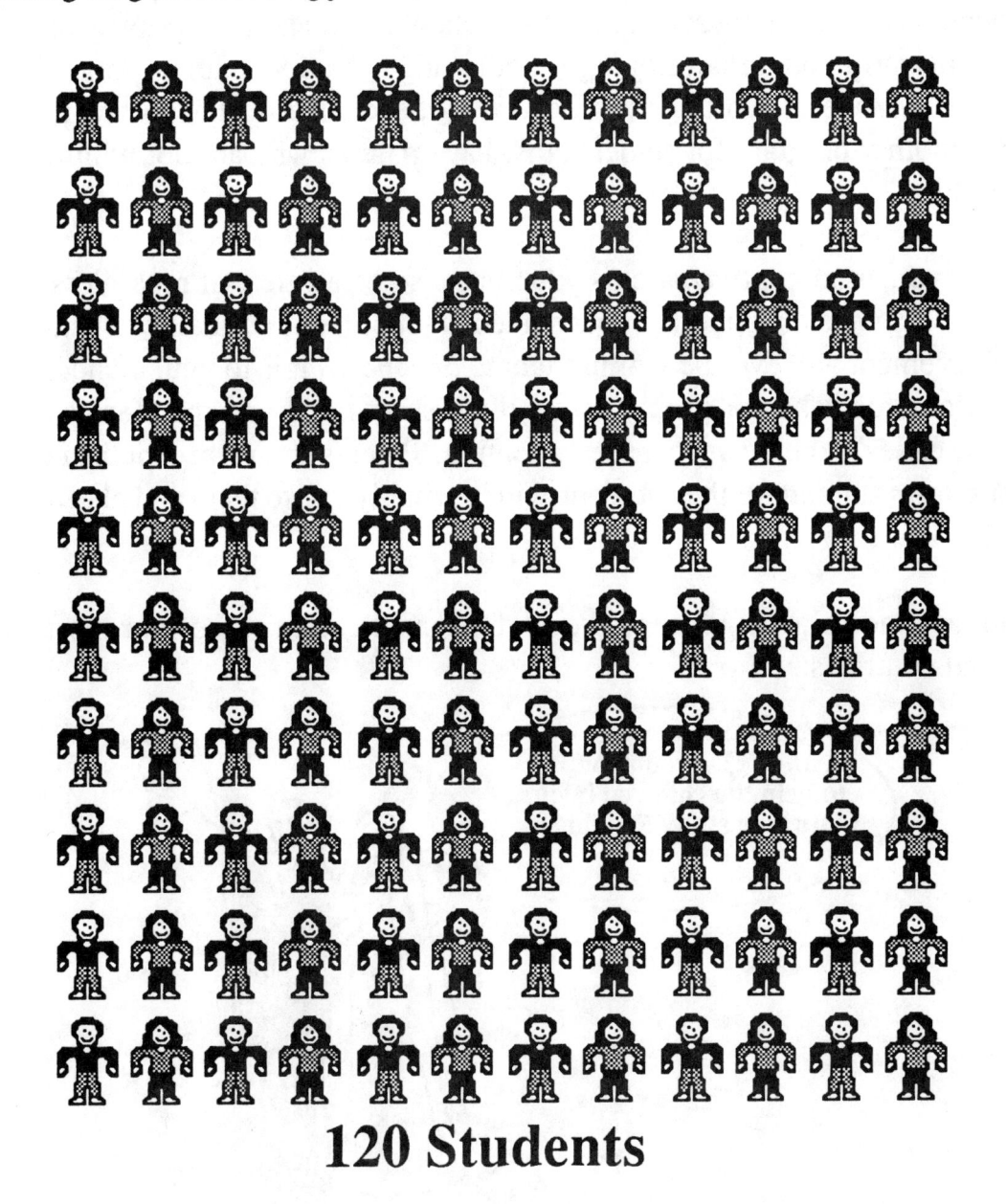

120 Students

As you know by now, our approach is to try to help kids survive in the present system. And the public system is unfortunately short-handed to do the job adequately. That's why we think this important job of shaping study skills is best accomplished by teamwork between counselors and parents. Improving study skills is more of a *behavior/follow through problem than a teaching problem*, although both are involved. If teaching students study skills were enough by itself, there probably wouldn't be a need for this book.

Given our current educational system, many, many students need **sustained, long-term support** (combining hard love and soft love) to benefit properly from their education. The best *practical* way of reaching failing students is to encourage school counselors to define school failure as a top priority and take **a leadership role** in developing school-wide behavior shaping programs for students. At least two kinds of programs are needed: those that involve parents, and another program for students that have parents who are not willing to be involved.

However, as supportive parents you must also be aware that regardless of the level of counselor support at your student's school, it is unlikely your student's achievement will ever be as important to *anyone* as it is to you. School interventions for behavior problems are often short-lived and there are constant "new crises" coming up that need attention. Parents should accept the fact that long-term support for their student will inevitably fall to them and plan accordingly.

Perhaps radical changes should even be considered in one of our most basic social contracts: (!)

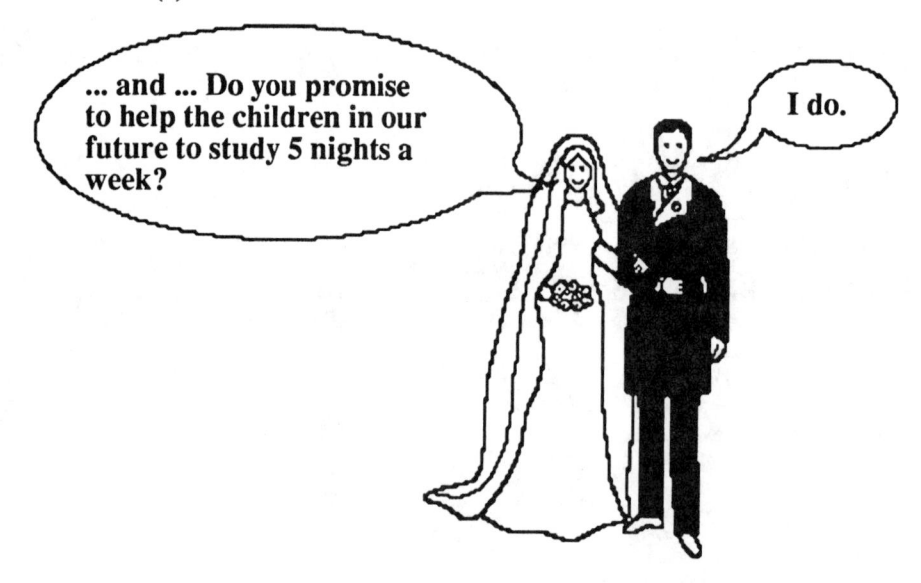

... and ... Do you promise to help the children in our future to study 5 nights a week?

I do.

Common Problems and Solutions

Problem 1: Your student is backsliding on keeping a logical notebook in which new papers are filed **every day** by date and section.

The Solution: First of all, don't underestimate how important this is. For some students, it is actually more important than the amount of time they study. Use a little trick daily that we learned from a girl who used to have this problem. After being confronted one week, she came back the next week, and showed me it was cleaned up by *holding her notebook upside down by the flaps* and letting the pages all hang down. **Nothing fell out!**

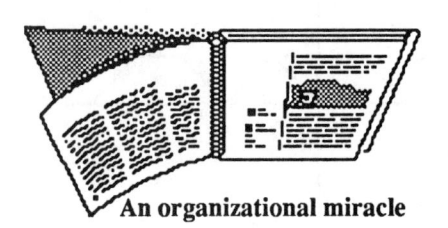

An organizational miracle

Give your student stopwatch time to clean up their notebook each night. They should *do this first,* before doing any other homework. You may even wish to enter it into the **Study Plan** like it was a subject.

Problem 2: The student is not yet studying as much as they need to.

The Solution: Add 10 minutes every week until you have established the minimum time the student needs to study each night. Remember, students can study more than this minimum when they need to.

Problem 3: The student still occasionally tries to convince you they don't have any homework.

The Solution: There is no such thing as not having homework. Learning never stops. What you are doing with the **Study Plan** approach is to budget your time. Consider the graph on the following page.

Cramming

Reviewing

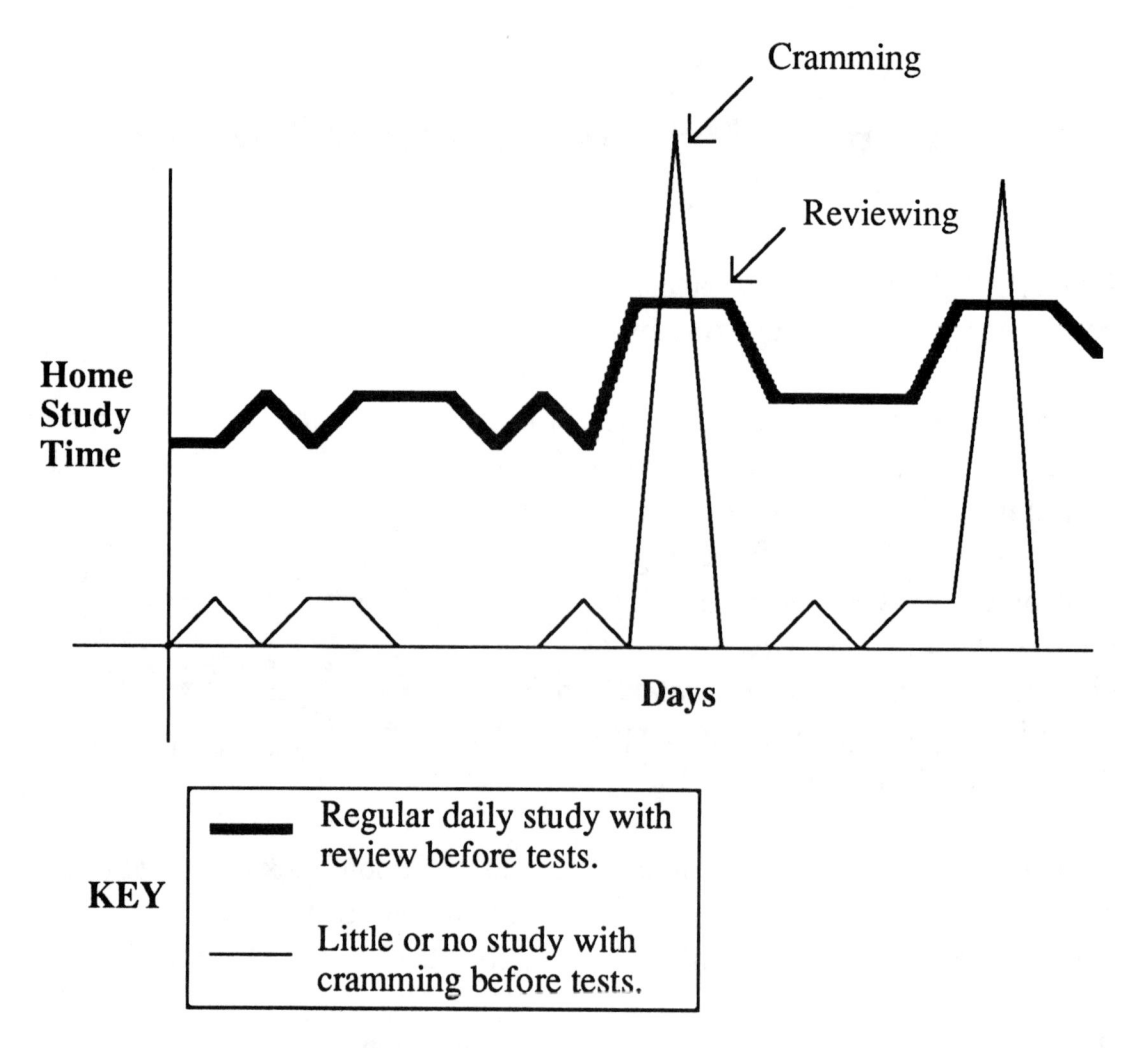

Home Study Time

Days

KEY

▬▬▬ Regular daily study with review before tests.

──── Little or no study with cramming before tests.

What you see here with the dark line is a student who keeps a *nice steady pace* of study activity going all the time. Notice that the time spent reviewing before a test is a little less than for the student who crams. This is because the student who keeps up every day **is not trying to learn all new information the night before a test.** Of course, students who learn to keep up every day also tell us they have less anxiety and fear at test time.

Follow the 3 rules:

1) The student may study ahead or behind in any subject and reread or rewrite any assignment.

2) If this is not enough, the student is to go back to teachers and politely inform they are trying to study each night and *could they please help them out.* Teachers are generally most willing to help and often come up with great ideas.

3) If neither of these two ideas is enough, the student is to check out 3 books related to their subjects from the library and read those during study time. **Parents can also assign specific work to build skills.** For example, when my daughter was in the second grade it was a rule that she worked on mastering math facts four nights a week.

The point is that you will never get on top of this problem unless you are consistent.

Study	Study	Study	Study	Study	OFF	OFF
Study	Study	Study	Study	Study	OFF	OFF
Study	Study	Study	Study	Study	OFF	OFF
Study	Study	Study	Study	Study	OFF	OFF

Next comes a section on why you need to **rewrite papers.**

Why Rewrite Papers

First let us show you a *great looking* first draft (even though some students think it looks like a chicken danced across the page):

The second draft looks like this:

Why Rewrite Papers?

Many students in public school have little idea why rewriting papers for school is necessary. It's to present their best work. Oddly, they don't think it will make a difference. They haven't yet learned that capable college students nearly always rewrite original drafts. The trick is to wait a day or two to go back and clean up unclear grammar or present ideas more logically. It becomes a matter of personal pride to write so precisely other people understand them easily. They believe it's up to them to communicate well, not to the reader to "divine" his or her meaning.

The final draft is on the next page.

Why Rewrite Papers?

Many students in public school have little idea why rewriting papers for school is necessary; it's to present their best work. Oddly, they don't seem to think it will make a difference. This is because they haven't yet learned that authors and other knowledgeable writers nearly always rewrite original drafts.

The trick to improving your writing is to wait a day or two, then go back to your draft to clean up unclear grammar or present ideas more logically. This way, you can "criticize" your own work before others do. In effect, you will raise the level of your writing one whole "notch" without knowing one thing more about writing than you do now.

Remember, it's up to you to communicate well, not to the reader to "divine" your meaning. Make it a matter of personal pride to write so precisely that other people understand you easily.

Special Assignment

This week you will have an assignment to rewrite a paper for one of your classes. The method you are to use is to **write on every other line** when you are doing your rough draft. Then write it over.

There are two reasons why you must write your rough draft on every other line. The first is that you will have plenty of "thinking room" between the lines to make corrections, the second is that it ensures you will rewrite it (you can't turn it in like that).

You do not have to rewrite your paper *twice* like we have done here, rewriting *once* will be sufficient. To help you remember to do this, you will be asked on your **Checklist** next week if you did it.

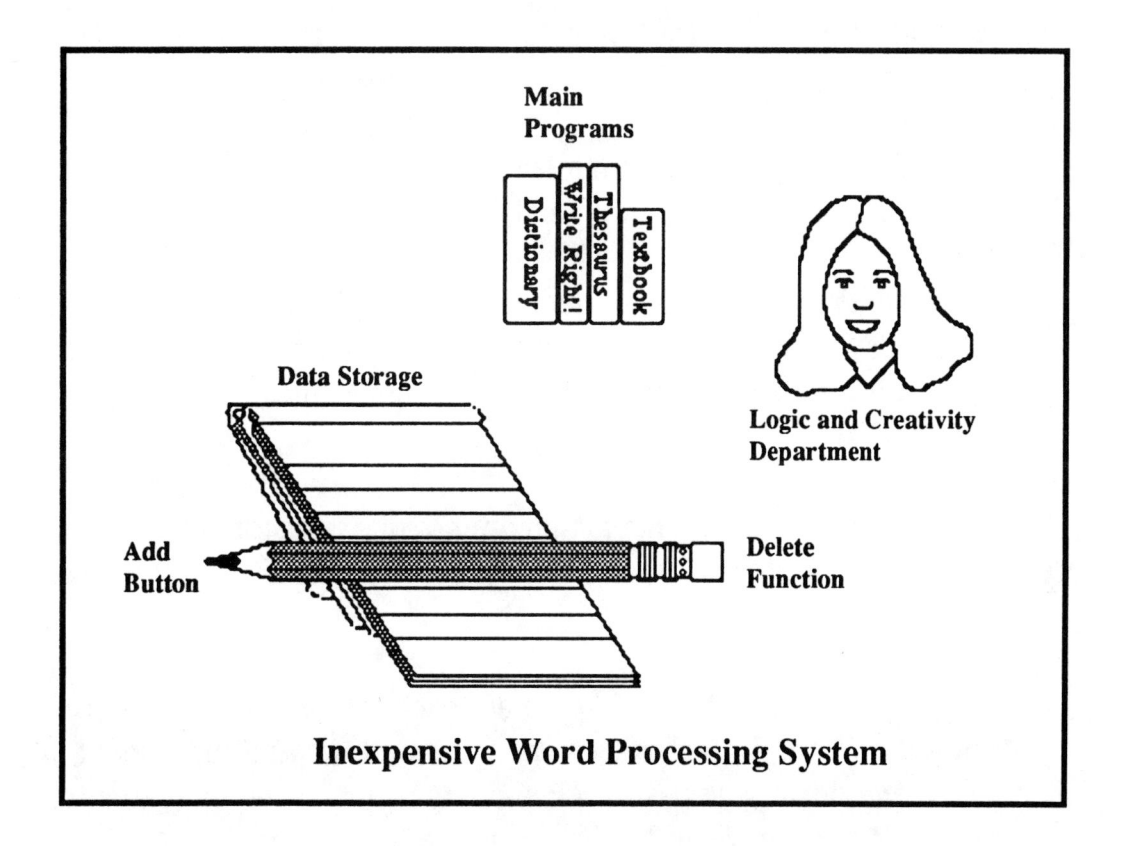

Inexpensive Word Processing System

- Main Programs (Dictionary, Write Right!, Thesaurus, Textbook)
- Logic and Creativity Department
- Data Storage
- Add Button
- Delete Function

Next is the Study Skills Checklist.

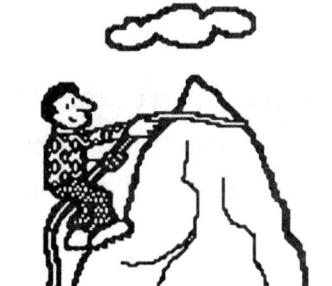

The Checklist

(Parent and Student do together)

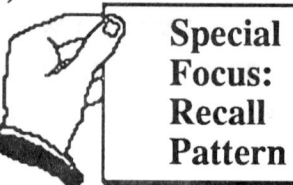

Special Focus: Recall Pattern

Mark the following **yes** or **no** as was true of your week.

___ **The student made a complete Recall Pattern.**

___ The student used the stopwatch and recorded accurate times at each study period.

___ The student is now using a standard 3 ring notebook with divider tabs. All sections are arranged in logical order by subject and date.

___ The student made his/her contracted study goal for the week or worked on Saturday morning until the contracted study time was made up. (Note: It is a parent responsibility to ask about this and to enforce it if necessary).

___ If the student has assignments that are not due immediately, he/she worked on them for at least 15 minutes each night or until they were done.

___ The student took the Study Plan to all teachers for comments once during the week. Low grades were compared with minutes spent on that subject during the past week and any needed time increases for next week were made and written into the Study Plan.

___ The student recorded every assignment, test, and quiz in the Assignment Sheet.

___ The student turned in every assignment this week.

___ The student took the Study Plan to his/her parent for their initials after every study period.

Next, turn to the **Study Skills Summary.**

Study Skill Summary
Parent and Student do Together

1) **Negotiate the amount of study time** and enter it on a new **Study Plan** (a new Study Plan and Assignment Sheet are at the end of this chapter). Put the new Assignment Sheet and Study Plan at the *front of the student's regular school notebook* and be sure all school subjects are listed on the new Study Plan. Have your student **record his/her study time every day.** Parent's initial the Study Plan. **Don't skip the initials!** If your student didn't bring the Study Plan to you to initial last week, ask to see it each night.

2) If your student procrastinates, set a time to begin and allow 15 minutes and ONE SECOND leeway, then **assign an extra 20 minutes of homework**.

3) See that your student has a **quiet place to study** at a table or a desk. No TV, no radio, no stereo, no phone calls during study time.

4) The student **must use the stopwatch correctly.** NO EXCEPTIONS.

5) Check and **initial the assignment sheet daily** if your student is having trouble turning in assignments. If your child loses the assignment sheet or the study plan, begin a new one the same day. NO EXCEPTIONS!

6) Once a week, make sure your student gets a **teacher signature** for each academic class.

7) If you need extra support, **make an appointment** to talk with a teacher, counselor, or principal.

THERE IS NO SUCH THING AS NOT HAVING HOMEWORK! The only students who say this are underachieving. Remember, the student can (a) study ahead or behind and/or rework assignments, (b) ask teachers for help and/or extra credit to fill up homework time, and (c) check out three books related to his/her subjects from the library to read during study time.

Parents may also know that the student needs to work on certain weaknesses and may assign the student a particular task. For example, parents may require their student to work on math facts, vocabulary, spelling lists, or independent reading.

Go over Your Checklist

Now, return to your Checklist on page 105 and make a plan with your student to correct any of the questions that were answered "no."

You should have already negotiated the amount of study time the student will study and the student should have **written it into the Study Plan.** If for any reason this hasn't been done, do it now.

You are now set for the coming week.

If either of you are even a little concerned that you may have a misunderstanding about your exact agreement, you may write your plan below.

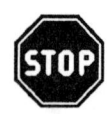

_____

_____

_____

_____

_____

This is the end of Week Six. On the next two pages are a new **Study Plan** and **Assignment Sheet.** You may use these this week but *do not* go to the next chapter, Week Seven, until you have studied for one week. However, do be sure to **plan** the day of the week you will read Week Seven and mark it on your home calendar.
See you next week!

Study Plan
Academic Skills Workshop

Name: _____

Date: _____

Daily Goals

Subjects:									Week Total	Teacher Comments: Grade/Attitude/All Work Turned In?
Total Stopwatch Time For All Subjects:									WEEKLY AVERAGE = _____ Minutes/Day (Add total number of minutes for the week and divide by 5 days.)	
When Did You Start?										
When Did You Finish?										
Place You Studied:										
Parent's Initials:										

COPYRIGHT © January 1, 1988 by Counseling and Workshop Professionals

Unauthorized Reproductions Are Illegal and may be Punishable by Large Fines.

Students who have individually purchased this book may make copies for their own personal use. Copies may not be made for friends. School Districts are **Expressly Forbidden** to replicate these materials. A special discount is available to schools. Call **(503) 588-1010** for ordering information.

Assignment Sheet

Write down the exact assignment before leaving class

Class	Assignment	Date Given	Date Due	Date Turned In	Parent Initials

Week 7

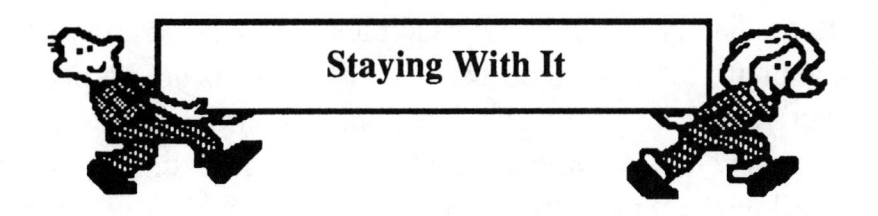

Staying With It

Staying With It

As you approach the end of the book, you may be wondering what's going to happen when you finish. Well, we hope that if you have come this far that you recognize that your progress came with effort and therefore it's real. However, there is also **real danger of backsliding** if you neglect the lessons you have learned. Fortunately, you now have the skills and structure necessary to help your student immediately should this happen.

We encourage all of you to continue using the stopwatch tool and do home recording. **If, and only if,** your student is now handling school to your satisfaction as a parent, you may discontinue the weekly feedback from teachers. However, at the *slightest hint* that things are not going well, start it up again. If your student is not yet taking care of school business almost perfectly, **continue to get feedback from teachers indefinitely. Period.**

Students vary greatly in the amount of support they need to continue. A relative few have immediately grasped the principles in this book and put everything into practice pretty much on their own. Most students are helped a great deal by a more active level of parent participation. It's hard to be specific, but when students keep up *good work habits* for about 6 months using the **Study Plan** we are ready to allow them more freedom in deciding how they will handle school. However, *they still must meet our approval.* Most teenagers are developmentally ready to organize themselves with adult direction; few are ready assume this responsibility completely. They do not have yet have the life experience and perspective to know what it means to work for a living. But when they leave home and life itself forces them to finish growing up, the **work habits they "had to learn" in school and at home, will be ready to help them like an old friend, even if the habits are not yet "perfect."**

On the other hand, those who have no history of working to achieve goals will find their late teens and early twenties filled with painful turmoil that has little direction and few reference points. When working behavior has become "automatic" for some, requiring no conscious thought or effort, others will have a serious life crisis and spend valuable time learning a myriad of little lessons about planning and followthrough. And this all takes place in the context of falling in love, marriage, babies, and coping with the necessity of earning a living. A little foresight can go a long way in life. Parents: your student still needs you to see ahead and pave the way into the future. The thanks you will get may not come for many years. If it's of any comfort, your children will almost undoubtedly experience the same thing with their future children, *just as you were probably not the most grateful of human beings* with your own parents many years ago when these issues were more personal to you.

Therefore, while you still have the time (and luxury) to shape behavior in your home, we would advise you to continue using the method you have learned for *at least* another 4 months. We think that many parents and students may choose to start at the beginning of this book and work through it again. What you are working toward is the time when **external structure has been internalized.**

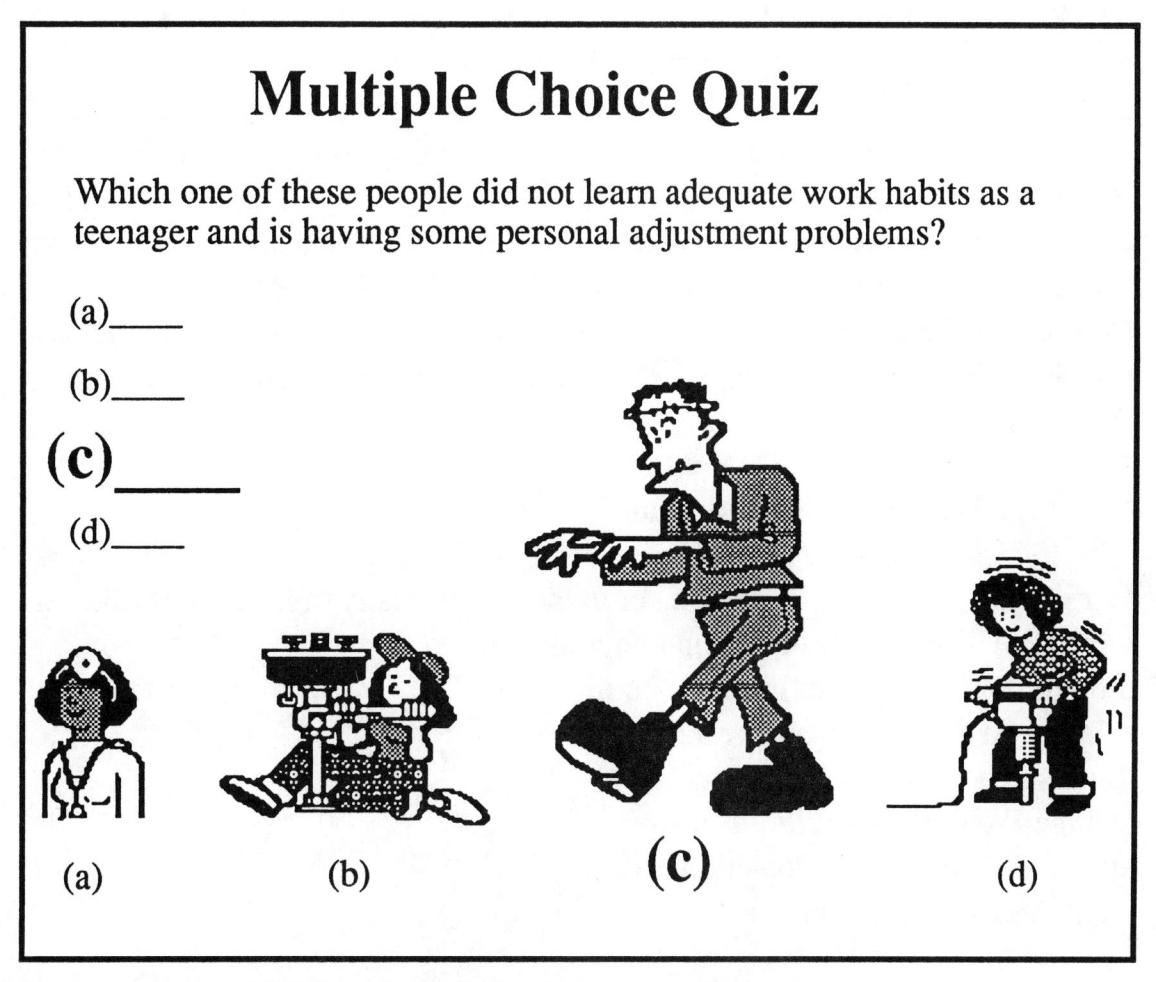

Multiple Choice Quiz

Which one of these people did not learn adequate work habits as a teenager and is having some personal adjustment problems?

(a)____

(b)____

(c)____

(d)____

(a) (b) **(c)** (d)

If you guessed **"C"** your insight is, in a word, awesome.

Next, read about **Closing the Loopholes.**

Closing the Loopholes

I never actually met Wendy. But her mother was in my office and she was crying hard. As the story unfolded I learned that she was a single parent and lived alone with her 14 year old daughter. They had been through years of very serious problems and this caring mother was feeling pretty hopeless. During the past week Wendy had been caught breaking into a house with some other kids (first offense) and referred to the Juvenile Department. Wendy got very angry every time her mother tried to talk with her about it and she "won" control each time because her mother would quit in frustration and tears.

As we talked further, it became clear that Wendy had been out of control for years. She was very good at manipulating situations, lied sometimes to cover herself, and pretty much came and went as she pleased. Of course, she was also absent from school most of the time. What interested me most about her school pattern was she had developed illness to a fine art to avoid being there. Typically, at her mother's insistence, she got out of bed in the morning and went. However, by about 10:00 a.m. most days she had such a bad headache or stomachache that she "just couldn't stay there." The school counselor would call her mother for permission to send her home and she would go back to her house. *Nobody knew exactly how she spent the rest of her day.* This had been going on for two years. In fact, it appeared that Wendy had worn down the school so much that her avoidant behavior really wasn't challenged very much anymore.

Getting a Handle on the Situation

Her mother, of course, had taken her to the doctor many times to see what was wrong. The doctor couldn't find anything and thought Wendy was not too ill to be in school. At first, her mother didn't think she had the strength to try to change Wendy's behavior. But she eventually helped develop and implement the following plan.

This may come as a surprise, but her problem isn't physical

First, we decided that we simply couldn't let her go home by forcing the school to make a phone call. It was too easy. Her mother decided that she would call her doctor to see if he would be willing to be the judge about whether Wendy was too sick to stay at school. The doctor was *pleased* to help. Next, the mother **made a commitment** that if her daughter said she was ill she would leave work, pick her up, and take her to the doctor. Immediately. The doctor's word would be final. No more would Wendy be in such easy control of the situation.

The next step was for the mother to go to the school with Wendy and explain this plan to the vice principal (we choose the vice principal because they are not generally known to be sympathetic with manipulative behavior). The vice principal was so enthusiastic about this plan that he even volunteered to take Wendy's temperature *before* he called Wendy's mother. That did it! Wendy wasn't about to let the man within 10 feet of her with a thermometer. The game was up, and she was *furious*. As they left the office, Wendy turned to her mother in a crowded hall, yelled an obscenity at her, and asked sarcastically if "she was happy now." It was very hard on the mother, but she stuck to her guns.

What happened next, as *a direct result of preplanned structure,* was that Wendy immediately began to **stay in school every day.** Furthermore, she eventually stopped complaining about being sick. She even started to do some work. Two weeks later her mother came back for a follow-up session. She was still worried about her daughter, but now she smiled with pleasure when she recalled how Wendy had told her she loved her this week for the first time in two years.

On Reflection: Although we hope you are not having problems of this severity, this story highlights several principles used throughout this book, .

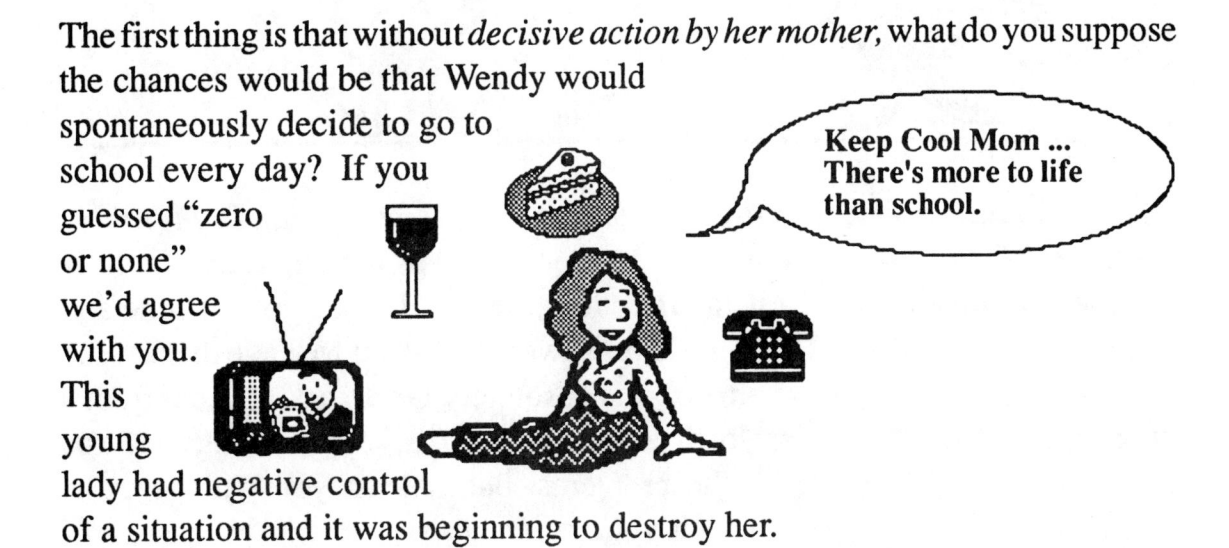

The first thing is that without *decisive action by her mother,* what do you suppose the chances would be that Wendy would spontaneously decide to go to school every day? If you guessed "zero or none" we'd agree with you. This young lady had negative control of a situation and it was beginning to destroy her.

Keep Cool Mom ... There's more to life than school.

The second point is that over a period of time she had built a "fool proof" plan to fail that was built on assertions that all the adults knew were "off the mark," but she convinced them to accept reality as *she* defined it.

The third point is that she took advantage of any and all loopholes. Pretending illness was her major method, but there were others. When we want to change self-destructive behavior in children, and gentler methods aren't working, we must *close all the loopholes.* This always means that you must *analyze the situation objectively* and decide what a reasonable person should be doing. Then you make *sensible* rules that are **consistently enforced.** Nothing causes acting-out children to gamble on bad behavior more than the thought that they might get away with it. It's very exciting.

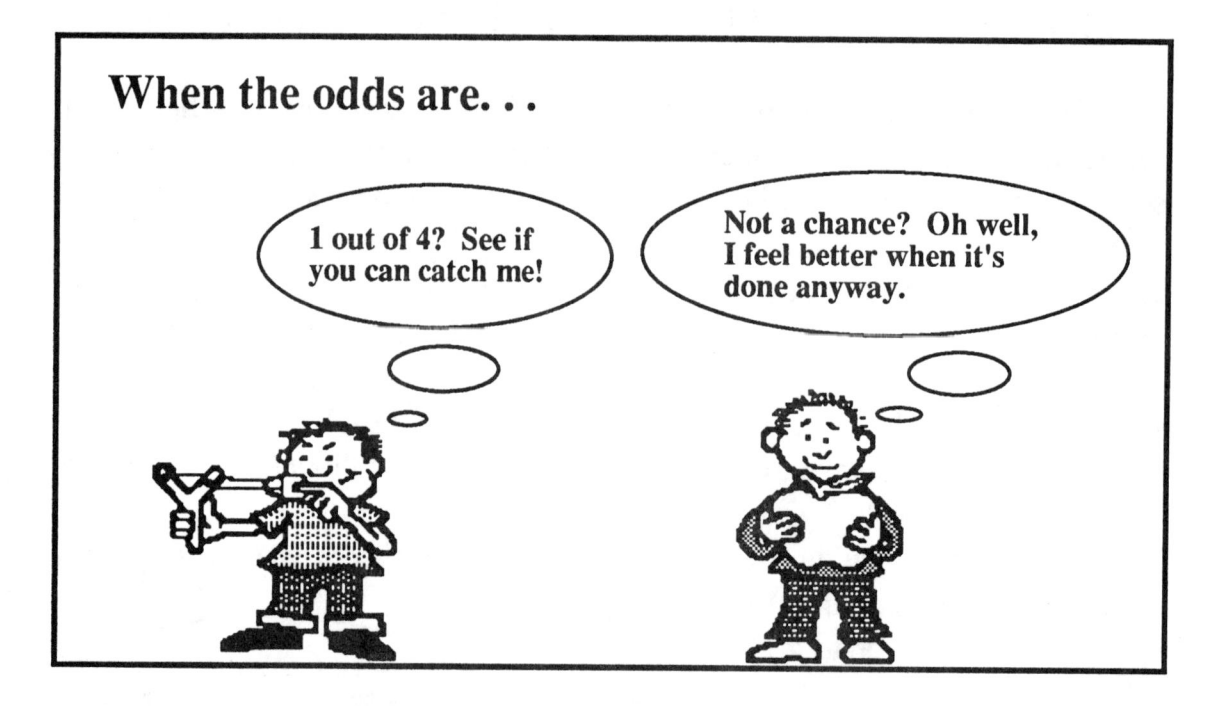

When the odds are...

1 out of 4? See if you can catch me!

Not a chance? Oh well, I feel better when it's done anyway.

The final point is that it *really does take a long time to change ingrained patterns.* Don't expect miracles to happen quickly. **Parents are the only people around who are in it for the "long haul."** It takes lots of time and energy to raise children. That's the bargain we make when we have them. But, when you get stuck (and we all do) it is absolutely OK to ask for help from a spouse, friend, teacher, counselor or support group. Just keep working on it. You may not be able to solve all the problems, but at least you will have the satisfaction of knowing you gave it **your** best.

(Has anybody out there guessed yet that one of my literary heros is Don Quixote?)

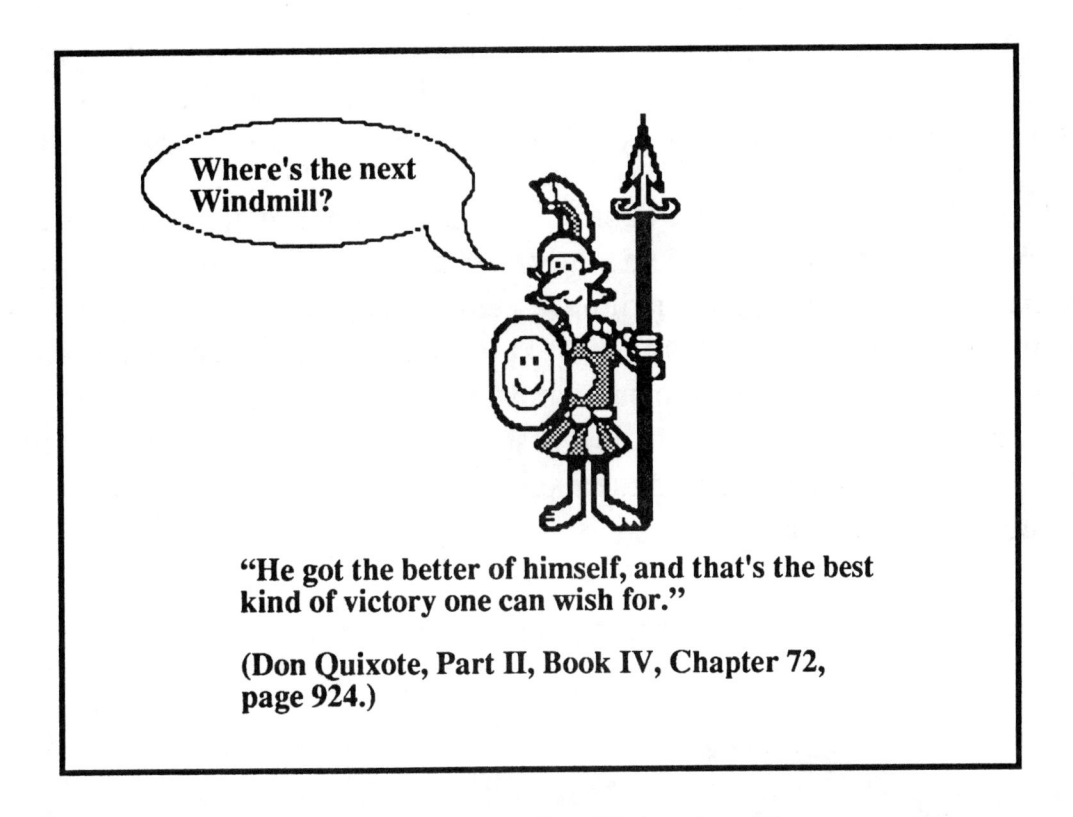

> Where's the next Windmill?
>
> "He got the better of himself, and that's the best kind of victory one can wish for."
>
> **(Don Quixote, Part II, Book IV, Chapter 72, page 924.)**

Common Problems and Solutions

Problem 1: The student gets telephone calls during study time and doesn't like it when you tell their friends they will call back.

The Solution: Just about everyone is conditioned to taking phone calls as they come in. However, calls *disrupt the flow of concentration necessary to getting good work done.* If you make this a rule and stick with it, the complaints will diminish in time, and your student's friends will learn when it's a good time to call. In fact, your student can simply tell them at school the times at which they will be unable to come to the phone.

Problem 2: The student has activities during the week and can't study every night they are supposed to.

The Solution: No problem. Simply study ahead earlier in the week. That is, if you usually study 60 stopwatch minutes a night and you want Thursday off, you could study 120 minutes on Wednesday (a day ahead) to clear Thursday for something special. Of course, **what you may not do**, is to promise to make up for Thursday *later* in the week.

Problem 3: The student understands about the T.V., but still wants to argue that listening to the radio or stereo during study time is really OK. Besides, they get nervous and may go crazy if they can't hear music while they are trying to think.

The Solution: For starters, we believe there have been *zero* admissions to State Hospitals anywhere in the United States over this particular issue, loud protests to the contrary. We repeat, radio and and stereo are **serious commercial business attempts whose purpose is to attract, and keep, your attention.** If they fail to do that, they will go out of business. In fact, high-priced specialists are often consulted about how to do it best. The solution is to *keep them turned off* during study time, and turn them on, *and enjoy them,* when study is over. Enough said, don't argue.

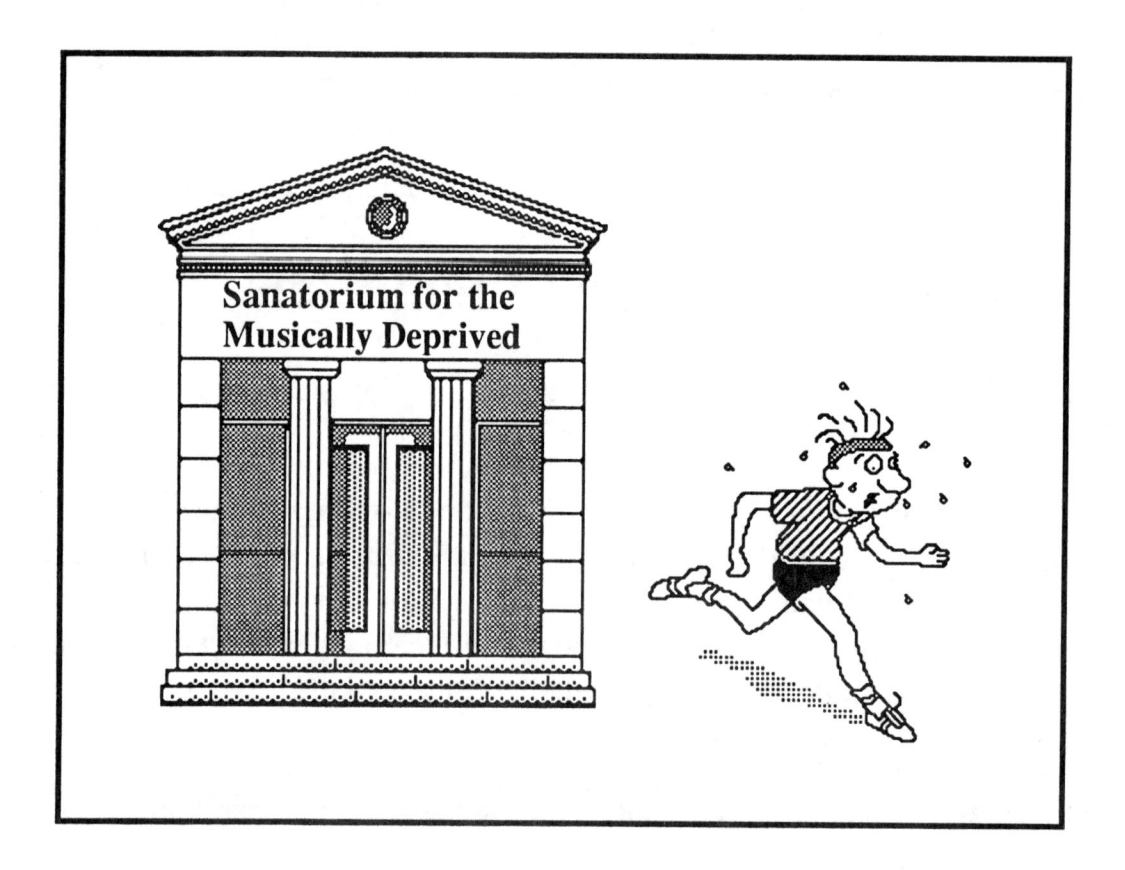

Next, **a few notes on notetaking.**

A Few Notes on Notetaking

Taking good notes is not terribly difficult but it does take self-discipline. For starters, it requires active attention to the teacher. The main thing is to capture the **key words** and **major concepts.**

At the beginning of each lecture, write the title of the lecture. Next record the day's date underneath it. From there, try to organize the concepts into an outline form, or use the "spider" idea of the Recall Patterns you have done. Don't try to take down *everything* the teacher says. Just try to get the **main concepts** and **key words.** If you use the outline form make your notes like this:

1. Main thought

    a) supporting thought
    b) supporting thought

We have found in practice that it may not be necessary to write the *numbers and letters* as long as you **indent** your supporting thoughts.

The better you get the lecture organized on paper the easier it will be to remember it later for the test. Be careful to get things accurately and leave yourself space in the margins to fill in material that your teacher **may give out of order.**

This relatively simple method will automatically help you to focus your attention in class. Don't hesitate to ask for a repeat of information or a clarification. It is common for speakers to talk faster than students can comfortably take notes.

Finally, feel free to develop your own shorthand. For example, I use s/o (someone), s/t (something), = (the same as), .. (therefore), and frequently omit vowels.

I bt u cn stl rd ths.

(I bet you can still read this.) After the lecture you can go back and fill in any unusual words that might get "cold" after a couple (cpl) days. Notes are intended to be a practical way to store information - not creations of great beauty. Start your own shorthand, stick with it, and watch how it grows.

> **Special Assignment:** Take careful notes in at least one class next week and show them to your parent.

The Checklist

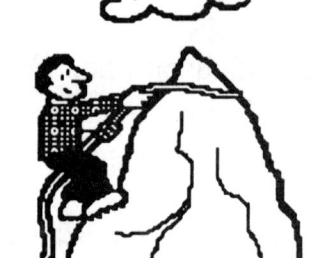

(Parent and Student do together)

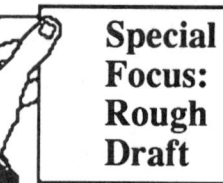

Special Focus: Rough Draft

Mark the following **yes** or **no** as was true of your week.

___ **The student rewrote a paper making a rough draft first.**

___ The student used the stopwatch and recorded accurate times at each study period.

___ The student is now using a standard 3 ring notebook with divider tabs. All sections are arranged in logical order by subject and date.

___ The student made his/her contracted study goal for the week or worked on Saturday morning until the contracted study time was made up. (Note: It is a parent responsibility to ask about this and to enforce it if necessary).

___ If the student has assignments that are not due immediately, he/she worked on them for at least 15 minutes each night or until they were done.

___ The student took the Study Plan to all teachers for comments once during the week. Low grades were compared with minutes spent on that subject during the past week and any needed time increases for next week were made and written into the Study Plan.

___ The student recorded every assignment, test, and quiz in the Assignment Sheet.

___ The student **turned in every assignment this week.**

___ The student took the Study Plan to his/her parent for their initials after every study period.

Next, turn to the Study Skills Summary.

Study Skill Summary
Parent and Student do Together

1) **Negotiate the amount of study time** and enter it on a new **Study Plan** (a new Study Plan and Assignment Sheet are at the end of this chapter). Put the new Assignment Sheet and Study Plan at the *front of the student's regular school notebook* and be sure all school subjects are listed on the new Study Plan. Have your student **record his/her study time every day.** Parent's initial the Study Plan. **Don't skip the initials!** If your student didn't bring the Study Plan to you to initial last week, ask to see it each night.

2) If your student procrastinates, set a time to begin and allow 15 minutes and ONE SECOND leeway, then **assign an extra 20 minutes of homework**.

3) See that your student has a **quiet place to study** at a table or a desk. No TV, no radio, no stereo, no phone calls during study time.

4) The student **must use the stopwatch correctly.** NO EXCEPTIONS.

5) Check and **initial the assignment sheet daily** if your student is having trouble turning in assignments. If your child loses the assignment sheet or the study plan, begin a new one the same day. NO EXCEPTIONS!

6) Once a week, make sure your student gets a **teacher signature** for each academic class.

7) If you need extra support, **make an appointment** to talk with a teacher, counselor, or principal.

THERE IS NO SUCH THING AS NOT HAVING HOMEWORK! The only students who say this are underachieving. Remember, the student can (a) study ahead or behind and/or rework assignments, (b) ask teachers for help and/or extra credit to fill up homework time, and (c) check out three books related to his/her subjects from the library to read during study time.

Parents may also know that the student needs to work on certain weaknesses and may assign the student a particular task. For example, parents may require their student to work on math facts, vocabulary, spelling lists, or independent reading.

Go over Your Checklist

Now, return to your Checklist on page 119 and make a plan with your student to correct any of the questions that were answered "no."

You should have already negotiated the amount of study time the student will study and the student should have **written it into the Study Plan.** If for any reason this hasn't been done, do it now.

You are now set for the coming week.

If either of you are even a little concerned that you may have a misunderstanding about your exact agreement, you may write your plan below.

_____

_____

_____

_____

_____

This is the end of Week Seven. On the next two pages are a new **Study Plan** and **Assignment Sheet.** You may use these this week but *do not* go to the next chapter, Week Eight, until you have studied for one week. However, do be sure to **plan** the day of the week you will read Week Eight and mark it on your home calendar. See you next week!

Study Plan
Academic Skills Workshop

Name: _____
Date: _____

Daily Goals

Subjects:						Week Total	Teacher Comments: Grade/Attitude/All Work Turned In?

Total Stopwatch Time For All Subjects:

When Did You Start?
When Did You Finish?

WEEKLY AVERAGE = _____ Minutes/Day
(Add total number of minutes for the week and divide by 5 days.)

Place You Studied:

Parent's Initials:

COPYRIGHT © January 1, 1988 by Counseling and Workshop Professionals
Unauthorized Reproductions Are Illegal and may be Punishable by Large Fines.
Students who have individually purchased this book may make copies for their own personal use. Copies may not be made for friends. School Districts are **Expressly Forbidden** to replicate these materials. A special discount is available to schools. Call (503) 588-1010 for ordering information.

Assignment Sheet

Write down the exact assignment before leaving class

Class	Assignment	Date Given	Date Due	Date Turned In	Parent Initials

Week 8

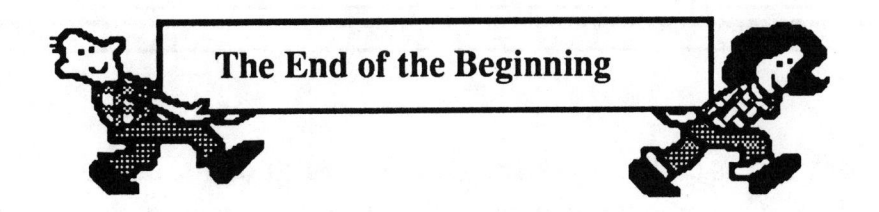

The End of the Beginning

The End of the Beginning

Please accept our **hearty congratulations** on making it to the end of the book! You have both worked hard and should allow yourselves the luxury of a pat-on-the-back. By completing this book you have demonstrated excellent persistence to task.

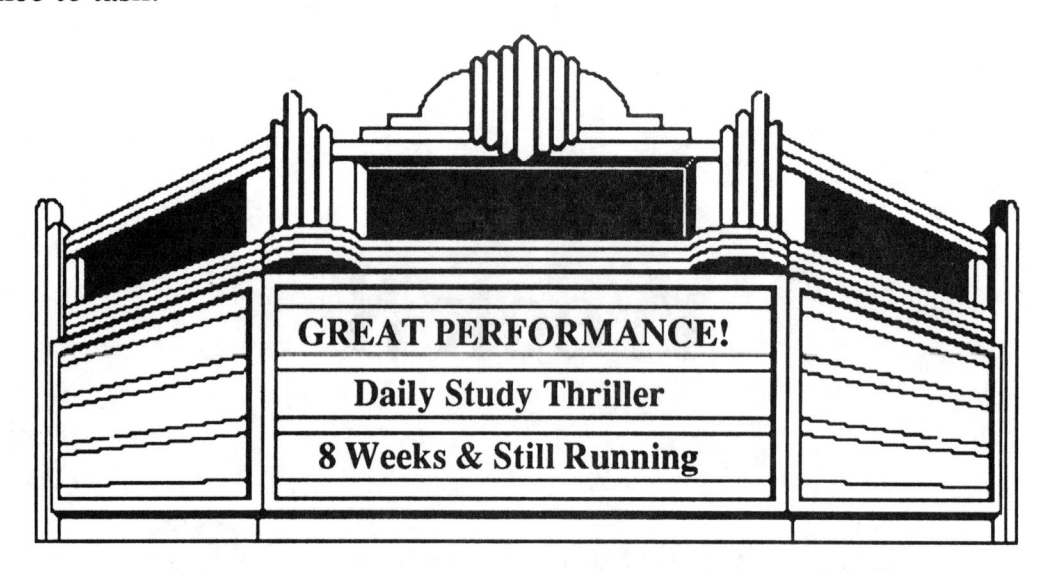

This kind of success calls for praise. Parents and students, take a moment here to go over the improvement you have both noted in the past 8 weeks. Sometimes it's easy to take it for granted. List 3 things that are better below:

1)_____

2)_____

3)_____

Since education is never really over, you will have more steps to take, but it should never be as hard as it was. By now, you probably have much better habits to help you and have finished the beginning stages of learning how to do it.

Next, read **Toni's Story.**

This story is not like the others. Some realities are harder to deal with than others. The young woman you are going to read about is doing something remarkable with her life. This is a true story, about someone who made so many awful decisions as a teenager it's a wonder she is still alive, let alone reaching for her potential every day.

This is also about education in the broadest sense of the word. We include it here as our way of saying to you that no matter how hard things get, **you must never give up.**

Toni's Story

Toni was an angry kid. To be more precise, an angry *defiant* kid. She had been abused and mistreated by many people and her trust level was rock bottom. By the time she was 11 she hated school so much she burned her school uniform in the gym. That finally got her expelled permanently, which was her goal. She didn't think she needed school and had been trying to get out for years. Her plan was to go to work and support herself. She didn't need anybody, thank you very much. The sixth grade was the last year it can be said she really attended school; she quit the pretense of going altogether in the 8th grade.

She moved out of her home and started living "life in the fast lane" in a large metropolitan city on the East Coast. Within a few years she was deeply addicted to drugs and was prostituting to pay for it. As her addiction hardened, she developed a dangerous intravenous cocaine habit. Her judgment was impaired of course, and she began to get arrested. Fortunately for her, she ended up in prison before the life she was living killed her.

In the relative safety of prison, Toni began asking for help which she often rejected. But even then, the urgency in her voice communicated a **desire to get better.** The **decision to get better** came shortly after she had run away from the prison release unit for the last time and come back after having been stabbed. Fortunately she was not seriously injured. But it shook her up plenty.

She decided to go to a residential drug and alcohol treatment center available only to inmates in the prison system. But when she made her appearance in front of the Board of Parole and Probation, she was told that her sentence was too short to be considered for this program. Toni told them she knew this was the case but was willing to voluntarily extend her parole date to go. Still, the Parole Board *ordered* her to go out on parole.

At this point, she did a very courageous thing; she told the Board she *refused to leave until she got the help she needed* because she knew she would be back without it. The Board asked her if she was aware that they could lengthen her sentence in prison if she refused a direct order. She said she knew that. Then the Board did the right thing and allowed her to go to the treatment program.

Toni emerged from that program 11 months later with a new attitude. She made the transition to a 12 Step self-help program as her primary support group and became an active member with a commitment to continuing recovery. Toni worked hard at everything she did to make it *honestly,* which meant, of course, minimum wage jobs. She even found time to volunteer to ring bells for the Salvation Army.

Things began to change for her. Instead of fighting against "the system" with all her strength, she joined it and *put her energy into growing.* She entered a community college and has proven that she has not only the self-discipline needed to learn, but also the curiosity and enthusiasm to stand out. She is known by her teachers and advisors as an exceptionally motivated student. And she does it in the roles of wife, mother, student, part-time employe, and practicum student. She is already making a respected place for herself in the helping profession, and in her second year of community college has made a long-range plan to get a Masters Degree in Social Work. She will make it.

Door to the World

For Toni, getting an education is the logical extension of all the hard work she did in therapy. After her marriage and family, education is the most important thing happening in her life right now. After what she has been through, she doesn't take it for granted. She has learned about personal integrity and responsibility; she works every day to act on those principals. As a result, doors are opening for her one after the other.

Next, learn about **Doing Your Best on Tests.**

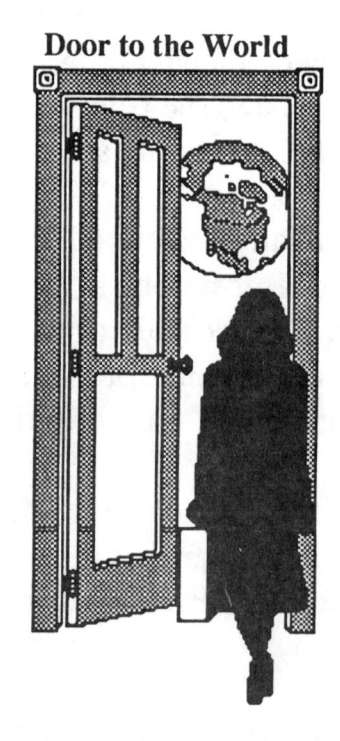

Doing Your Best on Tests

There are two main things to know about doing your best on tests. The first is that you must have started preparing for a big test days (even weeks) ahead. Cramming won't do it. The second thing is the strategy you actually use while taking the test.

Preparing Before the Test

1) Take class notes every day and start reviewing them *at least* 2 days before the test. Don't wait until the last minute! As you go over them, say the words out loud. Repeat hard words and concepts over and *over* and *over.*

2) Prepare the chapters you will be tested on with a **Recall Pattern** or **regular book notes.** To do your best it is strongly recommended you have the important facts *in your own handwriting.* You will remember more. Start going over your book notes *at least* 2 days before the test as well.

3) When you know you will have essay questions, write out 3 questions that you think *might* be asked. Next, with your book open, write out a "perfect" answer to each one and reread it until you know you will be able to remember it for the test. It is possible to get *very good* at guessing what might be asked. If you listen closely, your teacher might even tell you "between the lines" what will be on the test.

Strategy on Test Day

I've studied well and feel prepared ... I've studied well and feel prepared ...

When you go to class on test days, you will be understandably more anxious than usual. Get to your seat and take three deep breaths and loosen your muscles. **Do not talk with students about being frightened** by the test even if you are; that will only make you more nervous. Tell yourself the truth over and over, "I have studied well and feel prepared, I have studied well and feel prepared, I have studied well and feel prepared...."

When the test comes **read the directions carefully.** Next quickly read the test from beginning to end **without answering** any questions. There are two good reasons for doing this:

1) Human memory is built on a chain of associations so that when you remember one thing it often leads to another. As you read the test, you will prime the pump (your mind) with the subject vocabulary so that you will begin to remember things that were buried deep down. We have all had the experience of not being able to remember things that we immediately recalled after the test. The method of reading the test first will reduce this problem.

2) You need to find out which parts of the test are worth the most points so you can plan your time accordingly.

After you have read the test, go back through it and **answer the easiest questions first.** This works as a confidence builder and ensures that you will get credit for everything you do know for sure. Finally, go back through the test and work on the hard ones you are not sure about.

Remember:

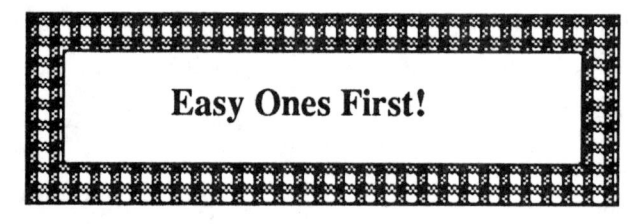

Easy Ones First!

Common Kinds of Tests

There are basically 5 ways teachers ask questions: True-False, Multiple Choice, Completion, Matching, and Essay. The strategy for each one is a little different.

1) **True-False Tests** are deceptively difficult. You must read them very closely. Often, just *one word* will make a critical difference. For example:

   a) Dogs **always** make good family pets. (F)
   b) Dogs **often** make good family pets. (T)

Beware of broad generalizations like *always, all, never, sole, none,* and *only* that imply there are **no exceptions.** These words often change an otherwise true statement into a false one. If you see these kinds of words, and you don't know the answer, mark the question FALSE. Also, **if any part of the question is false,** the answer must be false.

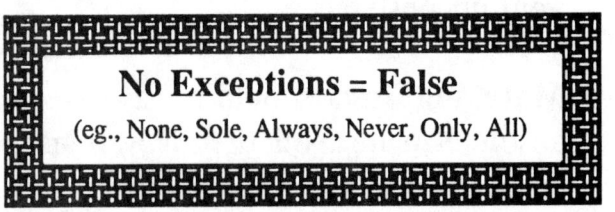

No Exceptions = False
(eg., None, Sole, Always, Never, Only, All)

On the other hand, when the modifiers imply there **are exceptions** with words such as *generally, usually, in most cases, probably,* and *often* the statement is more likely to be true. If you don't know the answer, mark these questions TRUE.

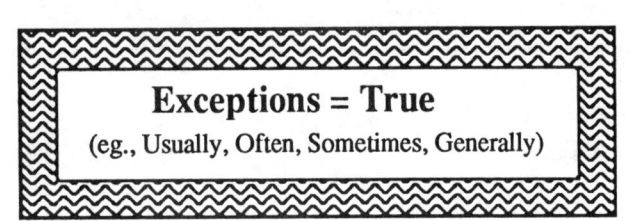

Exceptions = True
(eg., Usually, Often, Sometimes, Generally)

2) **Multiple Choice Tests** are designed to distract you from the true answer. The main thing here is to cross out as many of the obviously wrong answers with your pen/pencil as you can. This keeps you from involuntarily considering them with your eyes. For example:

   A student who has excellent study habits:

   a) always gets high grades in everything
   b) ~~is some kind of weirdo~~
   c) does school work carefully and turns it in on time
   d) ~~never has any time to play and have fun~~

We can easily rule out "b" and "d." With a little thought, you will realize that choice "c" is the correct answer.

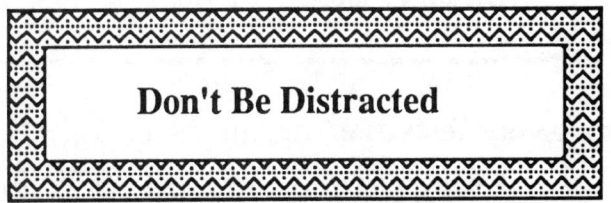

Don't Be Distracted

3) **Fill in the Blank Tests** are perhaps the most difficult. These are in the form of "George Washington spent a terrible winter at _____ _____ in which he lost many men to starvation and bitter cold." If you don't know the answer, read the question over several times and move on. When you have studied well the answer will

sometimes come to you later on as a "gift" from your unconscious.

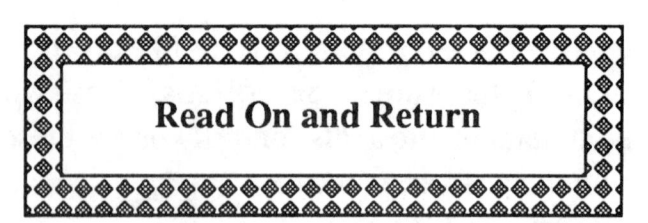

> **Read On and Return**

4) **Matching Tests** should always be done by matching the pairs you are absolutely sure about first. *Never* just go down the column in the order they come in because if you make an incorrect match, there will be only *wrong answers left* at the end. For example, you may be able to match all the dates below if you follow this rule, even if you don't know when Flag Day is. Try it.

Father's Day	March 17
Flag Day	2nd Sunday of May
Lincoln's Birthday	1st Monday in September
Valentine's Day	October 31
St. Patrick's Day	December 25
Mother's Day	4th Thursday of November
Independence Day	June 14
Labor Day	3rd Sunday in June
Halloween	February 14
Thanksgiving	July 4
Christmas	February 12

Answers:

Father's Day - 3rd Sunday in June, Flag Day - June 14, Lincoln's Birthday - February 12, Valentine's Day - February 14, St. Patrick's Day - March 17, Mother's Day - 2nd Sunday in May, Independence Day - July 4, Labor Day - 1st Monday in September, Halloween - October 31, Thanksgiving - 4th Thursday in November, Christmas - December 25.

5) **Essay Tests** offer the student the widest possible chance to pass or fail by his/her test taking ability alone. In addition, you will be graded on your writing skills, the way you organize (or don't organize), your handwriting, spelling, and factual presentation. For these kinds of tests, it is best to *think* before putting pen to paper. The easiest way to do this is to **brainstorm** on a piece of scrap paper before you start your answer. For example, let's say you are taking a test in a high social studies course and the question asks how you would explain the economic system in the United States to a foreign

131

exchange student. When you brainstorm, you should not be the *least bit critical* of the words you jot down in your list. You will go over this list later and pick out only those ideas you want to use. This technique works because words are *idea packages*.

A sample list for the question about our economic system might include words and phrases like:

capitalism	government social programs
inflation	government regulation
deflation	interest rates
money and banking	stock market
entrepreneurs	unions
competition	management
politics	strikes
federal reserve	lockouts
recession	profits
depression	corporate takeovers
trade deficit	security vs risk taking

Once you have this list, you can now think about how you want to begin your essay. In the actual writing of the essay, your opening sentence is probably the most important one because it defines the scope of your answer. Ideally, it should also engage your reader's curiosity to know more. The closing sentence is also quite important; it must summarize and end the essay in a way that feels logical and complete to the reader. By way of example:

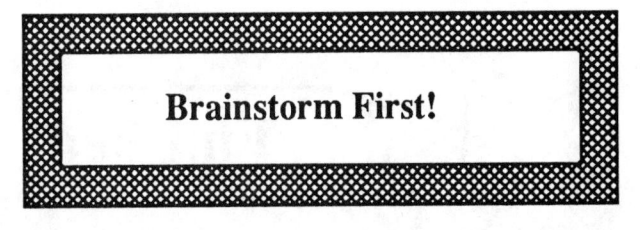

Brainstorm First!

One possible opening sentence: The United States economic system is a curious blend of fierce competition, near-monopoly control by huge private corporations, government regulation, and social welfare programs.

One possible closing sentence: Though it may be imperfect in design and seriously flawed by continual political compromises, it still fosters individual initiative and provides at least some aid to the less fortunate among us.

The Final Touches

It's a good idea to take tests with an erasable ink pen. Teachers like them because ink is easier to read than pencil and students benefit from being able to make changes and still turn in a neat looking paper. (It's well known among college students that typed papers get better grades on the average than handwritten ones because they *look better.*) Always go back through your work and look for misspelled words and other errors. It is common for students to unintentionally omit important small words so that a sentence may say "is" where you meant "is not."

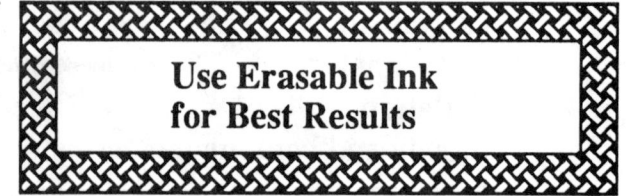

Use Erasable Ink for Best Results

After you have finished your final review, turn the test in and relax. It represents your best effort at studying properly, taking the test with care, and checking your work for accuracy. It should produce the best result of which you are capable. Nobody can ask for more.

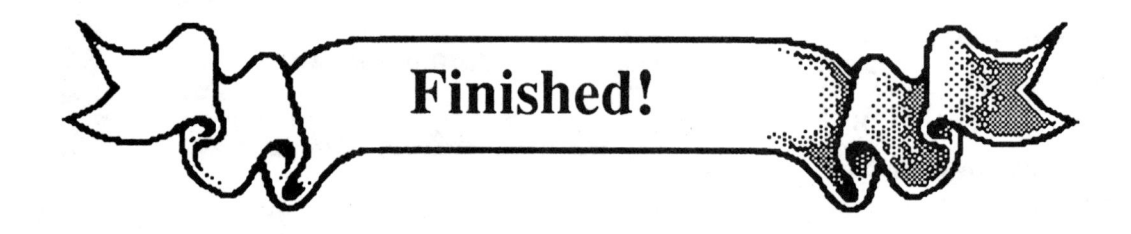

Finished!

Some Parting Thoughts

As we have written this book, Jerry and I have "replayed" countless discussions we have had with parents and students. Over and over we heard the same problems being anxiously discussed by parents and students from all walks of life - rich to poor and those inbetween. It appears that **underachievement has little respect for socioeconomic level or professional expertise** (we have had school teachers, principals, counselors and school psychologists in our Workshops). What all the parents had in common was a deep concern for their child's achievement and the motivation (approaching desperation in some cases) to try something new. We have witnessed some dramatic turnarounds and also had a few students who didn't respond. Most students studied longer, gained confidence, and felt better about themselves. Not everyone made large grade jumps, but many ended the workshop with improvements in one or two classes.

It is also safe to say that the great majority of the students experienced their parent's participation at the Workshop as an **act of caring about them** - even when they argued. We hope you have grown closer (in the soft love sense) as a result of doing this workbook together.

Where do you go from here?

The most important decision you will make tonight is whether to continue using the **Study Plan** or not. Frankly, we hope you will. It is a tremendous tool to help students become *more accountable* for themselves and it is a great aid in *diagnosing problem subjects* that are being understudied. It gives you and your student day-to-day concrete facts to talk about instead of the queasy uncertainty that most of you have dealt with before. It objectifies a parenting issue that can become *unbelievably complicated and emotional*.

And please don't forget that the **Assignment Sheet** is *absolutely essential*. As we have said, in some cases it is *more important* than the amount of time studied. Nearly all students who are getting "D" and "F" grades are following the royal road to failure: not turning work in. This common practice is totally unacceptable. Do not be swayed by arguments that "nobody else has to do this."

A realistic option...

... for many of you who have not achieved consistent performance yet is to start this book over and work through the chapters again, or at least continue on using the **Study Plan.** *It may be an excellent idea to do this together with a friend of the student and his or her parent.*

However, if you choose ...

... to stop doing the **Study Plan** (we hope you won't), then *the least you can do* is to set up a study time in your home and **be specific about the times,** for example, from 7:00 p.m. to 8:00 p.m.. Television, stereo, radio, and phone calls are not allowed. Above all, remember: **there is no such thing as not having homework.**

If you fail...

to make a plan, and *stick with it every day,* you will probably backslide quickly to the same place you were at before you started this book. We are **unconvinced** by *eager promises* to "do better on my own" until the student has demonstrated *complete competence* for at least 8 weeks by following a structured plan.

Promises, like new years resolutions, are usually made with good intentions, but are rarely sufficient by themselves to make permanent changes. Positive change that lasts *usually comes slowly.* And contrary to the hope many parents seem to have, it is not often the product of a single burst of insight. More often it starts with a dim awareness that a problem exists at all, and then slowly grows into a daily realization that the way you have been doing something no longer makes sense, though it may have at one time.

A WORD TO THE WISE

This book is all about improving performance. However, at some level, the implied message to children is that their performance is not good enough (why else are you doing this?). So, at some point **it is essential** that you allow your children to be **good enough.** They do not need to get straight "A's" or even a "B," "C," or "D" average to be perfectly delightful human beings. If your children do fail, it is important to love them, do what you can, and leave the door of hope open that in the future things may work out better. Don't forget there is a strong community college program in this country that allows some "forgiveness" to kids who were poor, even terrible students. It is a more risky path, but it does work for some who need to learn lessons the hard way.

There also seems to be a handful of people around who defy all rational explanation. They survive catastrophic childhoods and educational horror stories to grow into **extraordinary and talented** adults.

Our wish is for each student to fulfill his or her potential. Aim high, work hard, and **don't forget your obligation to give back something of value to others before your time on this planet is over.**

The End

(Did you remember to take notes in one of your classes? Appendix B contains an extra **Study Plan, Assignment Sheet, and Checklist** for those who want to continue using the tools now that they are done with this book. Individual parents who have purchased the book have our permission to photocopy these tools to use with your own children.

Appendix C contains advanced ideas to continue academic skill development.)

Appendix A

Certified Academic Skills Workshop Leaders

Oregon:

Monmouth-Independence

Jerry Gastineau (503) 838-0200

Portland

Glenn Rose, M.A. (503) 235-1529
Nonnie Wilson (503) 235-1529

Salem

Linda Bonham M.S.Ed. (503) 581-6025
Jerry Gastineau, M.S.Ed. (503) 588-1010
Dr. Ross Quackenbush (503) 588-1010

Stayton

Caroline Banks (503) 757-3449

California:

Kirkwood

Ron Salviolo (209) 258-8375

Petaluma

Julian Podbereski (707) 765-2034

Appendix B

Photocopy privileges of Appendix B materials are granted only to parents who have individually purchased this book. It is expressly intended that such photocopies be used only by the children of the parent purchaser.

SCHOOL DISTRICTS AND THEIR EMPLOYEES ARE EXPRESSLY FORBIDDEN TO COPY THESE MATERIALS. For information regarding training and discount rates to schools call Dr. Ross Quackenbush or Jerry Gastineau M.S.Ed. at (503) 588-1010. Please respect the many years of hard work that went into the development of these materials.

Study Plan
Academic Skills Workshop

Name: _____

Date: _____

Daily Goals

Subjects:						Week Total	Teacher Comments: Grade/Attitude/All Work Turned In?

Total Stopwatch Time For All Subjects:

When Did You Start?
When Did You Finish?

WEEKLY AVERAGE = _____ Minutes/Day
(Add total number of minutes for the week and divide by 5 days.)

Place You Studied:

Parent's Initials:

COPYRIGHT © January 1, 1988 by Counseling and Workshop Professionals
Unauthorized Reproductions Are Illegal and may be Punishable by Large Fines.
Students who have individually purchased this book may make copies for their own personal use. Copies may not be made for friends. School Districts are **Expressly Forbidden** to replicate these materials. A special discount is available to schools. Call (503) 588-1010 for ordering information.

139

Assignment Sheet

Write down the exact assignment before leaving class

Class	Assignment	Date Given	Date Due	Date Turned In	Parent Initials

The Checklist

(Parent and Student do together)

Mark the following **yes** or **no** as was true of your week.

___ The student used the stopwatch and recorded accurate times at each study period.

___ The student is now using a standard 3 ring notebook with divider tabs. All sections are arranged in logical order by subject and date.

___ The student made his/her contracted study goal for the week or worked on Saturday morning until the contracted study time was made up. (Note: It is a parent responsibility to ask about this and to enforce it if necessary).

___ If the student has assignments that are not due immediately, he/she worked on them for at least 15 minutes each night or until they were done.

___ The student took the Study Plan to all teachers for comments once during the week. Low grades were compared with minutes spent on that subject during the past week and any needed time increases for next week were made and written into the Study Plan.

___ The student recorded every assignment, test, and quiz in the Assignment Sheet.

___ The student turned in every assignment this week.

___ The student took the Study Plan to his/her parent for their initials after every study period.

___ When doing a writing assignment, the student rewrote the paper or making a rough draft first.

Appendix C

There are several advanced achievement ideas we promote with clients who have the energy and financial ability to go further. These are as follows:

1) Some things just never go out of style. A good vocabulary is one of them. If your children are headed for college they really should be working 10 minutes/night in a good **Latin/ Greek word root book.** It's interesting stuff. For example, *bio* (life) and *logy* (study of) = *biology* (study of life). Don't put it off until 3 months before the SAT test! We are talking **years** of patient work here. There are many sources to get word lists. I think all the study guides for the SAT test contain raw lists. A better resource are a pair of books by Luschnig, C.A. and Lushnig, L.J.: one is a textbook and the other is a matching workbook. You will have to order them from a good bookstore. They are listed in Books in Print. The titles are:

   Etyma: an Introduction to Vocabulary Building from Latin and Greek

   Etymidion: A Student's Workbook for Vocabulary Building from Latin and Greek

2) Another valuable little book is Write Right, by Jan Venolia. This is a handy, concise guide to grammar, punctuation, and style that covers the basics in easy-to-understand terms. Anyone who will write papers in college can benefit from this good book. Read about 2 pages at each study period until you finish the book. It's only 87 pages long. It's worth doing twice (or more).

3) For research-oriented students, Finding Facts Fast, by Alden Todd may prove useful. These are advanced techniques that are beyond the needs of most high school students. Mr. Todd has a background as a newspaper reporter.

4) Speed reading has probably been oversold yet it is a wonderful skill. Unfortunately the only self-help book I have seen that did an excellent job of teaching the techniques, Breakthrough: Rapid Reading, by Peter Kump is no longer in print. In larger metropolitan areas it is possible to find relatively inexpensive classes that teach it. By all means, take one if college is in the future. (If anyone out there knows a **good book** please send me the title.)

5) Last, but not least, we live in the **Age of the Computer.** Children who learn computer skills will prosper; those who don't will play "catch-up" as adults. The ability to type is **no longer a secretarial skill.** Computers are marvelous tools but they will not help those

who can only stare at the keyboard. *All children should be taught keyboarding* (the new word for typing as it applies to computers). We have noticed a great number of children getting "stuck" with hunt and peck systems because they are not learning early enough how to position their fingers. You should think about learning the keyboard as early as the second or third grade. With regard to computers you might think about:

a) Parents who are fortunate enough to afford a home computer should invest in one that will run educational software, **not games.** Computer games are a **repetitious waste of time and have addictive qualities** for some children. If you don't want to risk your child becoming a "computer junky" who spends hour upon precious hour trying to beat their old score we'd suggest you (a) don't have games in your home, or (b) set your trusty stopwatch to *strictly limit* their use (we are not aware of any ill health effects from doing this and your children will probably still love you in the long run).

b) **For the same reason that games are destructive, educational programs can be extraordinarily valuable:** many children will become absorbed in them for long periods of time. Educational programs often have an element of fun in them (which is wonderful). For example, we have a math program that speaks the words, "great job, your answer is correct!" each time my children do a problem right. They like it, and I think they learn more quickly than with flashcards and workbooks.

c) If computers are so great what kind should you buy? I'm pretty biased about this. For running educational software, Apple computers are so far in front of everybody else that there is no real competition. If you can afford the Apple GS, it's a very nice machine for students. If money is a real problem, check your paper for some good buys on the older (used) Apple 2c or 2e. Many people are upgrading their computers systems and are selling these older models cheaply. They still run very high quality educational software. These older machines have a good track record for durability so you will probably get years of good use out of them, especially if you by one that belonged to a family that didn't use it much.

If you really have a deep pocket and want something for yourself too, the Macintosh 512, Plus, and SE (also Apple products) are extraordinary machines that will do desktop publishing. Educational software is just beginning to be available for them. These are machines for creative people and will continue to grow in popularity. This entire book and 95% of the pictures in it were done on a Macintosh SE. My own children **assertively negotiate** with me for time on *my* "MAC" (they are more inclined to think of it as *our* MAC). This kind of "problem" is a blessing!

That about does it. If any of you have a favorite learning tool that is available on the market and you think others would benefit by using it, by all means send us a letter about it, or better yet, a sample. Happy Hunting!